50 Ways to Please Your Lover

THIS IS A CARLTON BOOK

Published in 2014 by Carlton Books Limited
20 Mortimer Street
London W1T 3JW

10 9 8 7 6 5 4 3 2 1

Text pages 6–13 and 18–54 © Susie Hayman 2000
Some of this material was previously published as
Pandora's Book in 2000, 2005.
Text pages 14–17 and 55–80 © Carlton Books 2009
Some of this material was previously published as
Fantasy Sex, by Lisa Sweet, in 2009.
Design © 2014 Carlton Books 2014

A CIP catalogue record for this book is available
from the British Library.

ISBN 978 1 78097 556 6

Printed in China

50 Ways to Please Your Lover

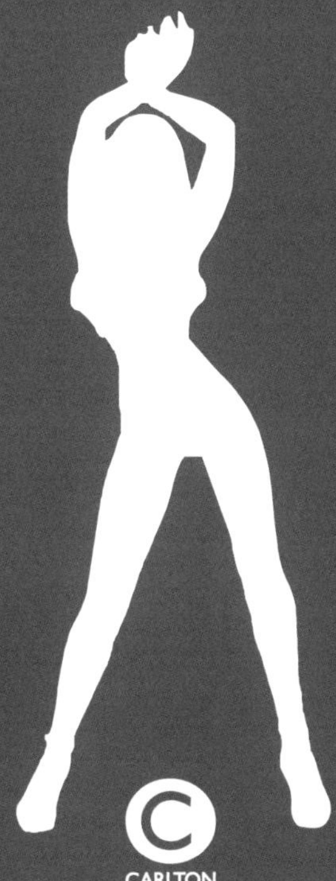

CARLTON BOOKS

Contents

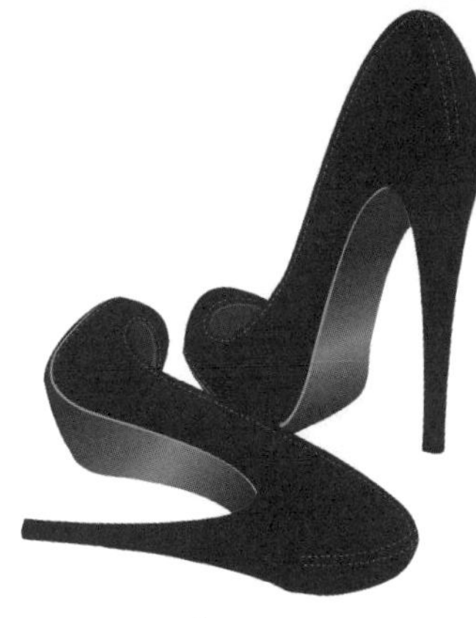

Further Roleplays

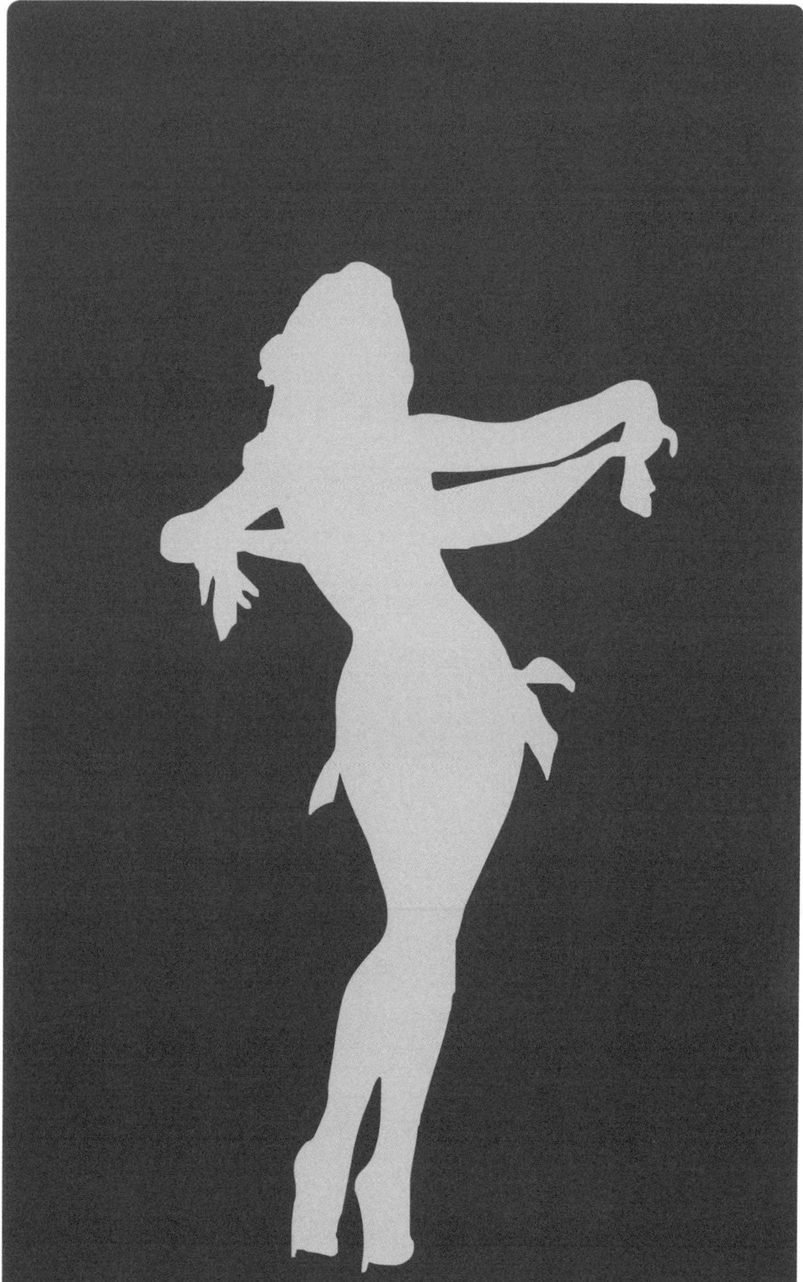

Introduction

SEX SHOULD BE FUN. OF COURSE WE HAVE SEX FOR THE SERIOUS BUSINESS OF HAVING BABIES AND FURTHERING THE SPECIES, BUT THE FACT IS THAT ON MOST OF THE OCCASIONS YOU MAKE LOVE, PREGNANCY IS THE FURTHEST THING FROM YOUR MIND.

You make love to express your feelings for your partner and to enjoy yourselves. It doesn't trivialize sex to acknowledge that; more times than not, fun and pleasure are the main driving forces. But there are two barriers to sexual bliss. One is a lack of knowledge: knowledge about sex, in general, and, in particular, about what turns you and your partner on. The other is the shyness and embarrassment; the wariness that has us holding back from doing the things we would really like to do with our partners. This book will be your gateway to a new sexual world together. Your new world will be one in which you can, and will, share knowledge, as well as becoming more confident, more knowing and far more sensually and sexually accomplished.

Most of us long for passion and romance. We want flirtation and fantasy, moonlight and roses. We want a relationship that has infatuation and excitement, lust and desire. We want to be endlessly surprised, to be thrilled and stimulated, both in and out of bed. We'd love to throw caution to the winds and fling ourselves into sexual adventures. We often don't, because we worry about what the neighbours will think, or are scared that our partners may be shocked. We need permission to give something different a go, and we need to know that what we'd like is normal and acceptable. And we'd probably appreciate a few hints on what we could try.

Open this book to set free a dazzling array of delicious ideas for any couple wanting to embark on new sexual adventures. You could be new lovers standing on the edge of a fresh love affair and wondering how far to jump in order to satisfy yourself and your new partner. You could be an established couple in a sexual relationship of months, years, even decades looking for new tricks for old dogs. Whether you're new or familiar, novice or experienced, young or old, straight or gay, you will find what you are looking for to put a kick in your love life.

Anyone can be a sexual adventurer – a pioneer of the bedroom, a trailblazer and explorer of the arts of the boudoir. We tend to think that the truly great lovers are people like Catherine of Russia or Don Juan; people who honed their flawless sexual technique with dozens of sexual partners. But being a good lover isn't about quantity, it's about quality. You can have plenty of notches on your bedpost and actually be terrible in bed if you assume that what works for one person at one time will always be sufficient or will have the same effect on anyone else. You can be the lover you've dreamed of being, and have the love affair to rival that of Antony and Cleopatra, Romeo and Juliet, Cathy and Heathcliff (but without the tragic endings), with just a little imagination and practice. There are two keys to sexual ecstasy, in knowing how to please yourself and set your partner on fire. The first is knowing yourself, and the other is being able to keep an open mind that is sensitive to your partner's responses.

Sex isn't something that you learn how to do in one night, on one sexual encounter. It's a perpetual journey of discovery where you can constantly learn new things and explore new places.

The sensual starting point for each lover is self-knowledge gained through self-pleasure. You don't have to understand the ins and outs of physiology to enjoy sex. Many people who write to me for advice worry about what they should be doing in bed to their partner, and what their partner should be doing to them. They ask for the definitive word on how to achieve sexual pleasure. If he twiddles this or she twitches that, if both fiddle about with the other,

would it result in rapture? The answer has to be "Well, sometimes, it depends." Because the real answer is that we're all different and what pleases you has to be something you and your partner find out for yourselves. The path to true sexual pleasure, as well as the path to true love, is one you have to travel for yourselves. It's a sensual journey of self-discovery and one you'll enjoy taking. The point is that you don't need to be told what should work for you – you are your own best experts. What you do need, perhaps, are some new ideas and the reassurance that it's OK to search. Most of us are surprisingly creative in our love lives if left alone to give it a go together. Social pressure can make us feel that sex is a taboo subject, a no-go area. What can set you free is communication. If you can be open with your partner about what you feel, what you need, what you'd like, and if your partner can talk to you too, intimacy can be that much better and put your sex life on a different plane. In fact, sexual experts are fond of saying that only 10 per cent of sexual excitement and pleasure is a result of what we do with our bodies. The rest is down to what goes on in our minds – our expectation and anticipation, our emotions and imagination. Sex is mostly in the mind, so developing this powerful tool in terms of sharing fantasies and role-plays opens up a world of sexual adventure that can make a couple's relationship dynamic and exciting. What this book will help you do is expand the potent force that is each individual's fantasy life, and help you bring this out to enhance your sexual relationship.

Using the ideas, you'll learn how to improve your loving communication. Understanding how to set the scene for a sensual experience can give you the impetus to add variety to your sex life together. But it also opens you up to feeling able to discuss your needs and desires, your fears and worries. The book will lead you, step by step, to unleashing the full power of your sexual and sensual imagination. You'll be surprised how inventive and downright extravagant you can be, once you know such behaviour is allowed and even encouraged between friends. One after the other, our scenarios will show you what is possible for lovers who would like to share a rich tapestry of new sexual adventures. You might think that the limit of what you can do in your love life is to slap on a bit of massage oil, lower the lights and maybe, just maybe, go crazy with a new sexual position or two. Once you've opened the book, the sky will be your limit, with exciting ideas and experiences for you both to pursue.

Having fun in bed does not mean being irresponsible or taking vows or commitments lightly. Respect and care for your partner are vital and basic requirements for any relationship, whether it's a new one that might not last long or an old one that has stayed the course. If you can't laugh and enjoy sex and come away from love making feeling better than when you started, what's the point? And there are so many ways you and your partner can liven things up, expand and deepen your intimate life together. You can dress for sex so that you excite your lover with your appearance – and undress for sex in ways that drive them wild. You can add the use of sex toys into your sexual repertoire – creams and oils, vibrators and dildos, straps, feathers and dice. As you further develop your sexual confidence, you can experiment with all sorts of sexual positions and exotic sexual variations.

Above all, you can develop and take pleasure in your sexual fantasies. We all have sexual fantasies. They may be thoughts and wishes that pop into your minds and play themselves out without any conscious control, or they may be full-blown sexual dramas that you make up deliberately and which proceed as you plan. When you have a sexual fantasy, you're using the largest sexual organ in your body – your brain. Knowing how to use it best is the key to a happy sex and love life. Fantasies should be fun. There's nothing weird or unusual in having them or using them to enhance your love life. Not only do most of us have sexual fantasies, most of us have similar ones. The 12 fantasies outlined in The Cards and in the first section of the book are a dozen of the most common. That isn't to say your dreams aren't your own and unique. But it is to reassure you that you're neither strange nor odd in finding these thoughts and ideas exciting, sexually arousing and stimulating.

The important point to note about fantasies is that they aren't real. But having

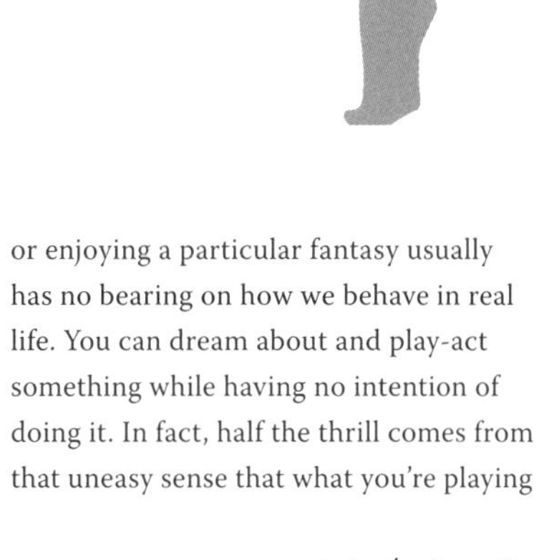

or enjoying a particular fantasy usually has no bearing on how we behave in real life. You can dream about and play-act something while having no intention of doing it. In fact, half the thrill comes from that uneasy sense that what you're playing about with is unacceptable, to society as a whole or to you in particular. This is why so many people find themselves drawn to sexual fantasies that seem strange or worrying. Imagining having sex with someone your own gender, or having your partner take you by force in spite of your protests, are both very common sexual fantasies – from people who would not welcome a same-sex relationship, and would hate to be taken against their will.

It's nothing to worry about if you find yourself having such fantasies and taking pleasure in them. Simply enjoying thoughts like these doesn't mean you will want to put them into action. Of course, drawing the line and recognizing the boundaries are important. To be able to enjoy this book to full, glorious and satisfying effect, you and your partner should know the difference between fun and harm, love and abuse, mutual pleasure and exploitation.

The key to acting out fantasies and letting your imagination loose is to set the scene. You can – and should – improvise and be spontaneous. But feeling confident enough to throw your inhibitions away and immerse yourself in the play often depends on doing your homework first. If you can arrange the room and your props and have the story and some of your lines agreed and clear in your minds, you'll find it surprisingly easy to let rip and become different people. By reinventing yourselves and your relationship, just for a short time, you can take back to your partnership and your everyday relationship a whole new fresh perspective and some invigorating ideas.

"YOU CAN DREAM ABOUT AND PLAY-ACT SOMETHING WHILE HAVING NO INTENTION OF DOING IT"

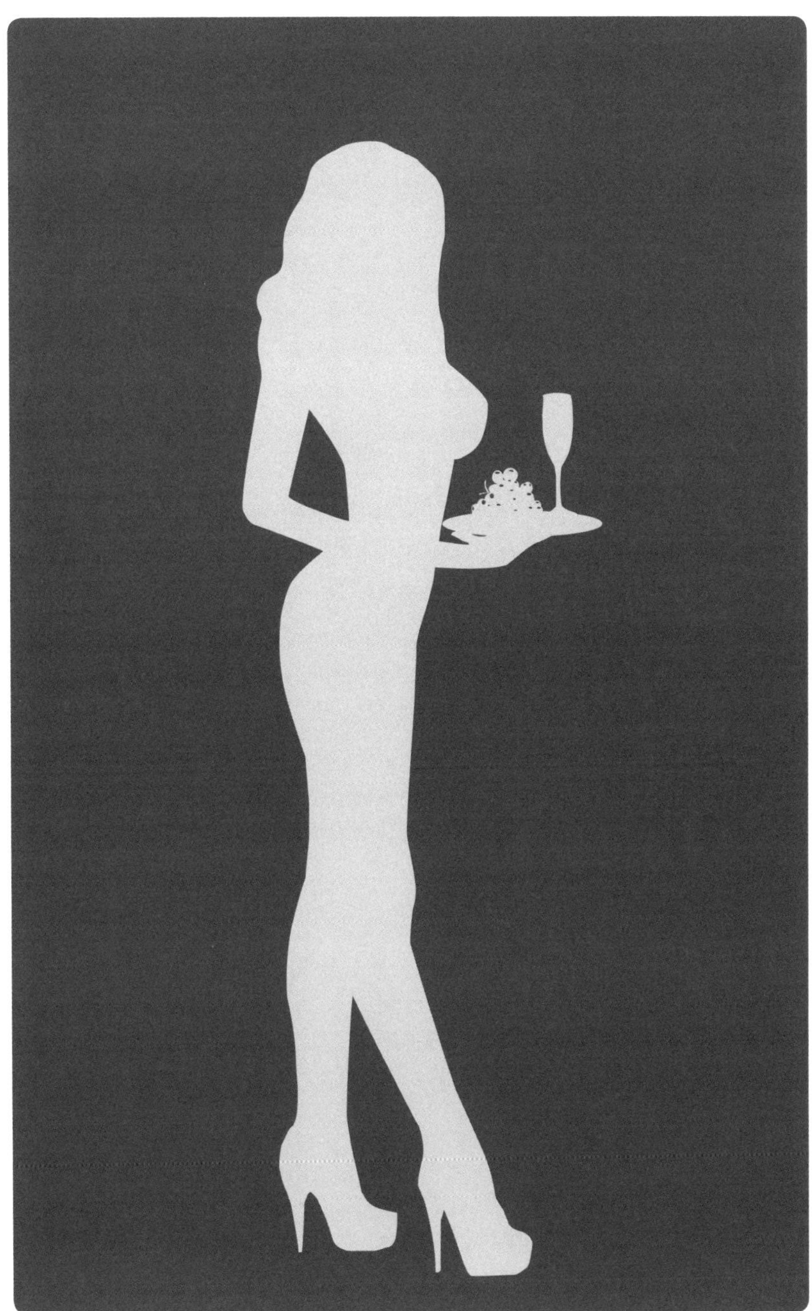

Top 10 Tips to Please Him

1

Men like their foreplay hard and heavy. So make him drool with these five lip-licking smack downs.

- Tug his bottom lip with your teeth
- Lightly suck his tongue when it's in your mouth
- Nibble at his neck
- Tickle the roof of his mouth with your tongue
- Cup his head and pull him toward you to deepen the kiss.

2

You don't even need to touch him. Just seeing you do some sexy thing injects an instant shot of testosterone into his bloodstream. Put him on guard by locking eyes with him. Then reach under your shirt, arch and unclasp your bra. Wriggle it free and toss it toward him. He'll be all over you.

3

Go ahead and bring him to the brink. Then ignore him. It's a guaranteed way to send him into a frenzy... and swell his orgasm later.

4

The small dent just above the crease of the bottom (aka "the sacrum") is absolutely packed with sensitive nerve endings. Use your fingers to rub its surface and around its edges. The harder the better, so don't be afraid to put your whole body into it.

5

The inner thighs are ultra-quivering to touch. They're also the home of the lymphatic system, which releases chemicals that cleanse the body of toxins. This is why kneading a handful of the soft flesh in this area can create a pleasant buzzy state.

6

Using both hands, start at the hips and caress the flesh, working your way toward the inner thighs. Now trace the same line with your mouth. Repeat this alternating sexy build-up until he can't take it any more (you'll know when this is because he'll push your head toward a more central between-the-legs region).

7

Give his tootsies a soaking by gently sucking the toes, from the big one down to the little one. Finish with a tongue swirl over the hyper-responsive in-step.

8

With your mouth around his penis, tickle his balls with one hand, using your other hand to scratch his inner thighs or stroke his bottom.

9

Feverishly flicking your tongue along his raphe (the vertical line in the middle of his scrotal sac) will send an electric volt through his system.

10

Play with his prostate and watch him prostrate himself before you. Hard to reach, this internal walnut-size gland is a pleasure minefield. Wrapping your lips (and hand, if necessary) around the shaft of his penis and, rather than doing your usual up-and-down thing, moving it toward his body will treat him to an inner massage.

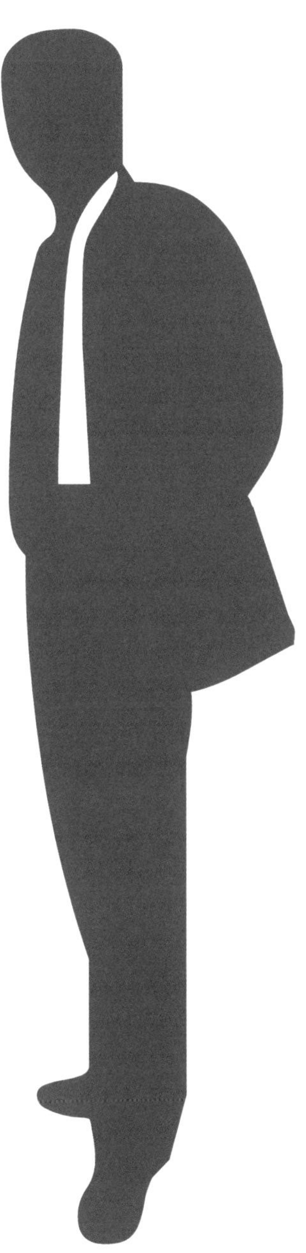

Top 10 Tips to Please Her

1

Find the pulse point (around 1¼ in / 3.5 cm under the earlobes and just under the jawbone) and, using three of your fingers, rub tiny circles with very light strokes. If you're doing it right, you should feel her pulse start moving faster than a train.

2

The area between the belly button and pubic bone is packed with pleasure points. To arouse them all, massage, lick or nibble the soft skin from the navel down to where the pubic hair begins.

3

The clitoris is a very sensitive soul, so switch between rubbing, stroking, licking and sucking, varying the amount of pressure you apply.

4

Dribble warmed-up (finger-test the temperature first) honey, chocolate or syrup over her body and lick off.

5

Gently pull back the labia as if you're opening curtains so that her entire love region is exposed. Now work your thumb and tongue over and under and all about.

6

Remember that there is so much more to breasts than the gumdrops on the top. Caress and lick the sensitive top, bottom and sides of her breasts before coming in for a nipple landing.

7

Lightly tap with your tongue or finger on the top of her clitoris while caressing the top of her bottom where the crease ends.

8

Turn your penis into your eleventh finger.
Grasp it at the base and slowly rub it over
her clitoris. At the same time, reach behind
and work your fingers against the rim of each
other's rear entries. Bliss off!

9

Give her a full working over inside, outside
and through the back. Begin with a sweet
circular stroke to her love bud. Once she's
feeling fine, crook your forefinger into a
"come hither" position and slip it inside
of her to tap lightly against the G-Spot.
While tapping, substitute your tongue
for the finger working her genital blossom.
This frees up that hand to gently rotate
around her back garden.

10

Instead of working her clitoris in an up-and-
down motion, trace around it as if you were
drawing an "8" over and over and – mmm –
over. By constantly varying the degrees
of pressure between hard and soft, you'll
soon put her into a layback spin.

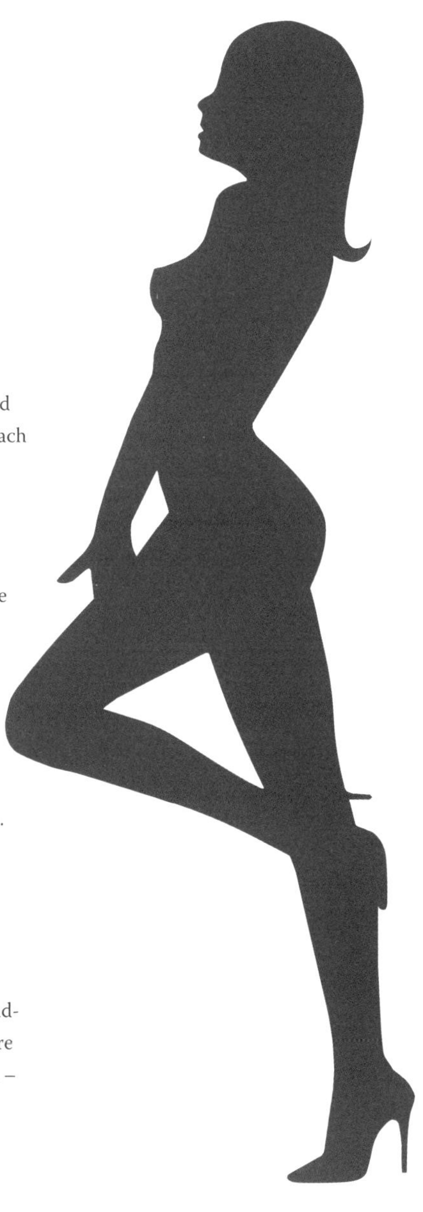

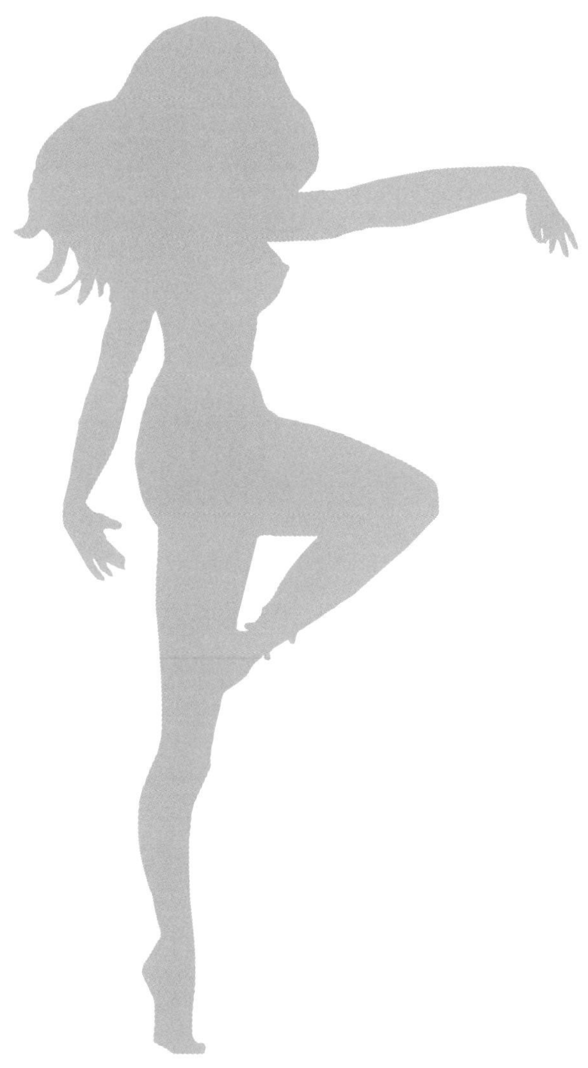

1
Virgin Nights

THERE'S NOTHING QUITE AS EXCITING AS
FIRST-TIME SEX. AS A TEENAGER, TAKING THOSE
ORIGINAL STEPS FROM HOLDING HANDS,
TO TENTATIVE KISSING, THROUGH TO PETTING,
YOU WOULD HAVE BEEN IN AN AGONY
OF UNCERTAINTY.

The mixture of terror, curiosity and anticipation made your pulse race and your stomach churn and it would have added to your sexual arousal. All that adrenaline racing round your body would have joined with those teenage hormones, to make first-time sex thrilling enough to have you coming almost as soon as you touch. There's still an enormous mystique attached to taking someone's virginity. Both men and women can be ecstatic at the thought that they might be their partner's first lover, the one who introduced them to the world of sex. Even if you've known your partner for years, you can recapture that kick by playing Virgin Nights.

One of you is going to be an innocent. Whoever picks the card is a virgin, or you can toss a coin to decide which of you will be the seduced and which of you will be the seducer. The winner puts themselves in the shoes of a school pupil stirred by the first glimmerings of sexual curiosity and desire. Our virgin is a stranger, so far, to shared bliss but not a total newcomer to the sensual pleasures. He or she has discovered the delight of self-pleasuring and so is all the more ready to be initiated into the world of adult sex. They've fumbled around with someone their own age a few times, but that seemed clumsy and unexciting. They've had "crushes" on film and pop stars, and have had quite a few sexual fantasies about them. Recently, our young virgin has been having even more explicit daydreams about a particular friend of a brother or sister. The other one will play this person – an older friend of a brother or sister. You're sexually experienced, confident and good-looking. You've met the young innocent before but never really noticed them. You're calling round to see your friend, with nothing on your mind.

Set the scene by arranging cans of soft drinks, schoolbooks and a teenage magazine around the living room. Put some music on, or turn on the TV or radio to something a teenager would watch or listen to. The virgin should be dressed in school uniform – a plain skirt or trousers, a white blouse or a shirt with uniform-style tie.

Start the action by imagining that the virgin has come home from school to find the house empty, parents and older brother or sister out. They're just about to settle down to homework or a coffee or soft drink when the doorbell rings and it's that friend of the brother or sister, dropping round to see them. The virgin invites the older friend in for a coffee, feeling both tongue-tied and thrilled. The rest of the family won't be back for ages, so here's a chance to have this sophisticated company for themselves. As well as having set the scene and imagined the state of mind of both the participants, have a few lines of dialogue prepared. Start off with the virgin telling the older friend, "They'll be back soon. Why don't you wait? I'll get you a coffee or a drink." Wherever the friend sits, the virgin then tucks in close – sharing a sofa or balanced on an armchair seat. The older friend isn't exactly averse to being sociable, either. There may be an age gap, but it's very flattering when you realize that an attractive, nubile-looking youngster is making eyes at you.

The older friend starts off being polite, asking about school studies and kindly enquiring what the young person hopes to do when they leave school. But then they pick up one of the magazines and realize that sex figures greatly in these. The teasing then becomes more explicit – "So this is the sort of homework you do, is it? What about the practical, how much of that have you done?" Lifting the drink, the older friend accidentally-on-purpose spills some on the uniform shirt.

"Hey, I'm really sorry. I'm so clumsy. You'll have to take that off or it will stain and you'll get told off. Here, let me

TOP TIP

We tend to imagine that when a virgin is seduced by an expert, it's a girl being won over by a man. One of the most potent myths, for both men and women, is of the older woman, a Mrs. Robinson, who will take a young lad in hand and lead him to manhood by teaching him some tricks. Add an extra boost to your love life by playing this one with her in charge.

help you." Riding over any protests, the older friend unbuttons the shirt and tugs it out of the waistband. By now you are up close and personal, and the older friend leans in and takes a long, lingering kiss. "Well, here's your chance to get a few lessons ahead." The older friend then offers to throw the dice to find the lesson for the day, and show the virgin how to do it.

Playing Virgin Nights allows you to remember what first excited you about sex, in general, and your partner, in particular. You might find yourself recollecting a particular sexual position, a particular sexual sound, a particular texture, article of clothing, scent or taste that lit you up the first time and still has the power to do it for you. You may not be able to bring it to mind just by thinking, remembering or reminiscing. Act it out and it may all come flooding back, with dramatic effect. This Virgin Nights scenario is only a suggestion. Think and talk about it, and it's probable that you and your partner may find a whole play in your own imagination, from your own memory, that you'd like to rerun or reinvent for your very own private Virgin Night. Many people, for instance, had their first sexual experience in the back or front seat of a car. If you have a garage or parking space that isn't overlooked, you could replay the end of the date that was your first time.

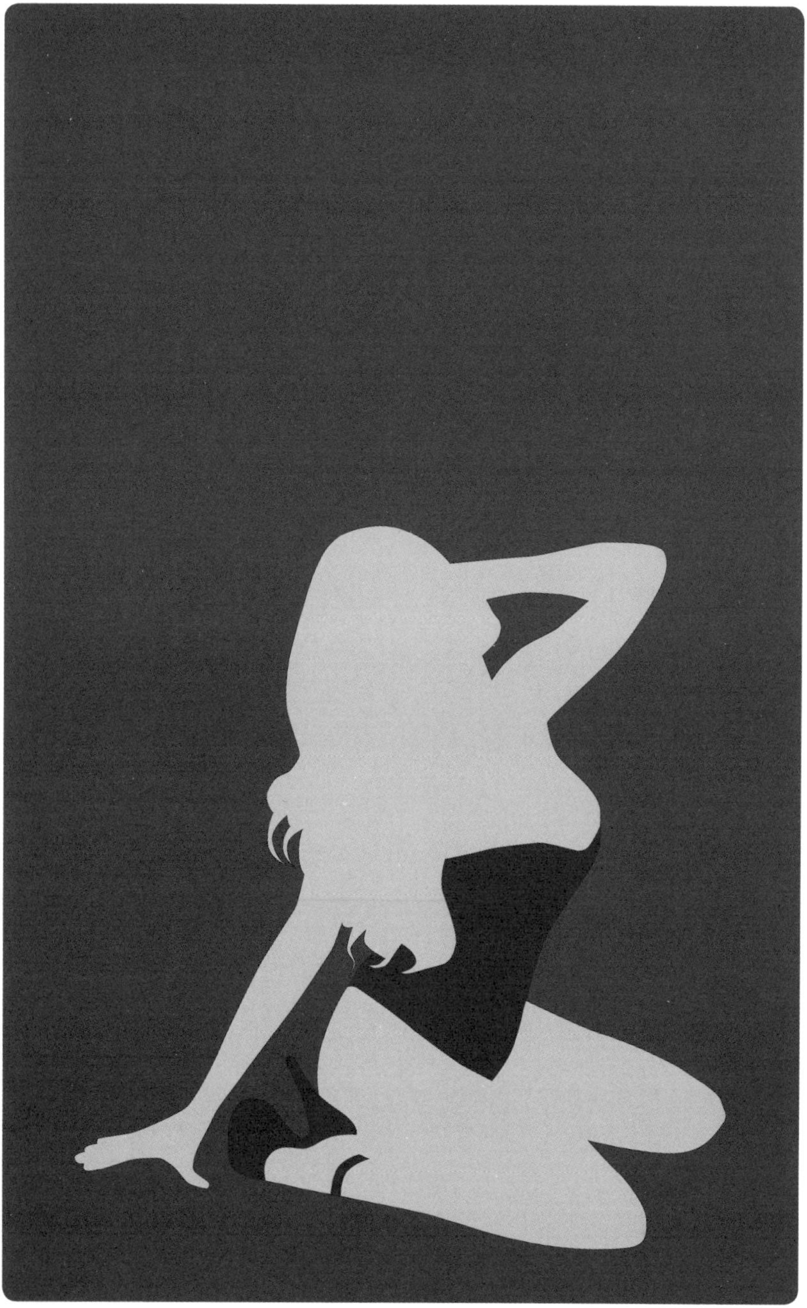

Exotic Erotic

HAVING SEX SOMEWHERE DIFFERENT, FOREIGN OR EVEN OUTLANDISH IS A FAVOURITE DAYDREAM FOR MOST OF US. THE REASON IS THAT BEING AWAY FROM HOME OFTEN RELEASES US FROM STRESSES AND RESTRAINTS.

It works in reality, when you go away on holiday. When surrounded by strangers with none of the friends, family or neighbours to tut-tut and carry tales, many of us throw away our inhibitions and act in ways we'd never dream of doing at home. We get drunk, dance on tables, fall in love with and make love to people we've only just met. But it's not just a question of not having to worry about a reputation with no prying eyes to see. It's also because we feel reality has taken a holiday, too. Back home, you wouldn't just be afraid of what people would think or say, you'd be scared of consequences. On holiday, you tend to feel they don't exist – as if a pregnancy or a sexual infection won't know where you live once you've gone home! Another reason is that we tend to feel they do it differently and far more sexily abroad,

so throwing caution and inhibitions to the winds is only following local customs. You can use all of this to cut loose in a sexual fantasy. Most of us need a way of feeling permitted to access our deepest, most secret and passionate desires. Imagining yourself in your dream place, far away from home and all its restraints, can do the trick. Your personal fantasy could be a Caribbean beach, for example. Set the scene by arranging plants and vases of flowers around the living room to mimic the jungle edge. Turn up the heating, and if you've got a sunlamp, switch it on. Lay out a beach towel on the floor or over a sofa in place of a sun lounger. Set a Piña Colada or other exotic drink by the side, with a bowl of exotic fruit, a bottle of suntan lotion and a feather. Dress yourselves in brief swimming gear – a bikini for her, a they do the same to you. You could use dialogue you've agreed before, or improvise as you like. Perhaps she says, "There's no reason to even keep our things on – here's the chance to get an all-over tan." He says, "Sure, but I've got bits that have never been seen by the sun. If we're going to lie here naked, that means we need to make sure every last inch of skin is covered and protected by suntan lotion."

Spread the suntan lotion all over each other, making sure to pay attention to every last bit. You'll raise the temperature if you give each other a running commentary as you do it, saying exactly where you intend to rub the cream and where you think you still need to be covered. "You need some here, on your nipples. Is that OK? Let me just smooth some here, on the inside of your thigh – am I tickling you?" Don't forget the cold drinks and fruit, laid temptingly near by. One of you could take a drink to cool down, and trickle a little on your partner's belly or cleavage. "Here, this will cool you down," you could say as you lick it off. The contrast between the heat and the cold can have parts of your body stand up to attention. Or you could cut open a peach and let the juice drip down your partner's legs, and clean it off with your tongue. Or slowly drop grapes, one by one, into your partner's open mouth. Imagine you can feel the heat – pretend it's almost too hot to do anything as energetic as make love. You might tickle each other with a feather, found on the beach. But mostly it's better, surely, just to smooth on the cream and lie there, enjoying the scenery. But as you stroke

thong for him. Close your eyes and imagine you've flown out the previous night and have just woken up in Paradise. You've wandered out of your luxury hotel room, strolled down the beach and have found a private area, obviously set up for your delight. You are sitting in the shade of the palms when you realize you're the only people there. You could almost believe you're castaways, shipwrecked on a deserted island.

Start the action by offering to spread suntan lotion on your partner, asking that and caress each other's bodies, the fact that there is no one else in sight means you can fulfil a lifelong wish – to make love on the sand. "Did you know," she could say, "that in some places it's considered really bad luck to make love indoors? Outdoor sex is the only acceptable way, so we're only doing what everyone else does."

If your fantasy place is a snow-covered chalet in a mountain retreat with a roaring log fire, lay out a shaggy or fleecy rug in front of your heat source. Make up mugs of creamy hot chocolate, and have some lotion on hand "to drive away the chill." Set the scene – you've just come in out of a blizzard, frozen to the bone and in wet clothes. "The best way to warm up is to strip out of these, and rub each other all over with a nice, warm towel. You'll catch your death if you don't get some feeling back into those toes. Here, let me rub some lotion over you to bring life and feeling back into you." You'll need to strike and stimulate every last centimetre of skin to make sure every bit is safe, and spill warm chocolate on each other to make sure that you're toasty warm. "Is this bit still frozen? Just show me which bits on you are still in need of being warmed up."

Bring the exotic to life and into your home by conjuring up unfamiliar scents and flavours. If you're setting the scene on a desert island, burn some flowery or spicy incense. Mix up the sort of cocktail you only drink on holiday – a jug of Sangria, a tall glass of Tequila Sunset or Rum Punch. If it's a mountain lodge, burn pine or cedar wood and drink Glühwein, hot chocolate or hot buttered punch.

"IMAGINE YOU CAN FEEL THE HEAT"

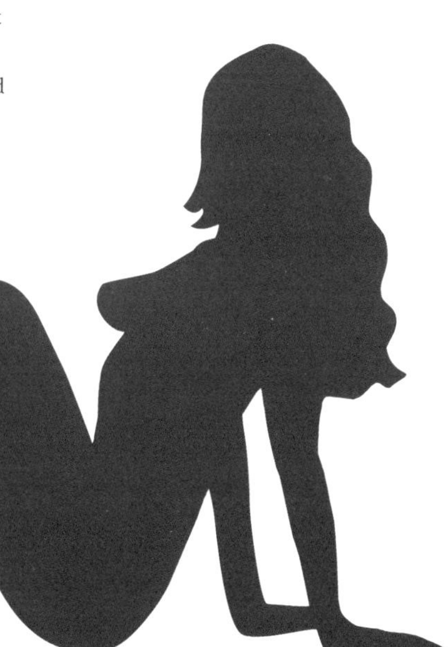

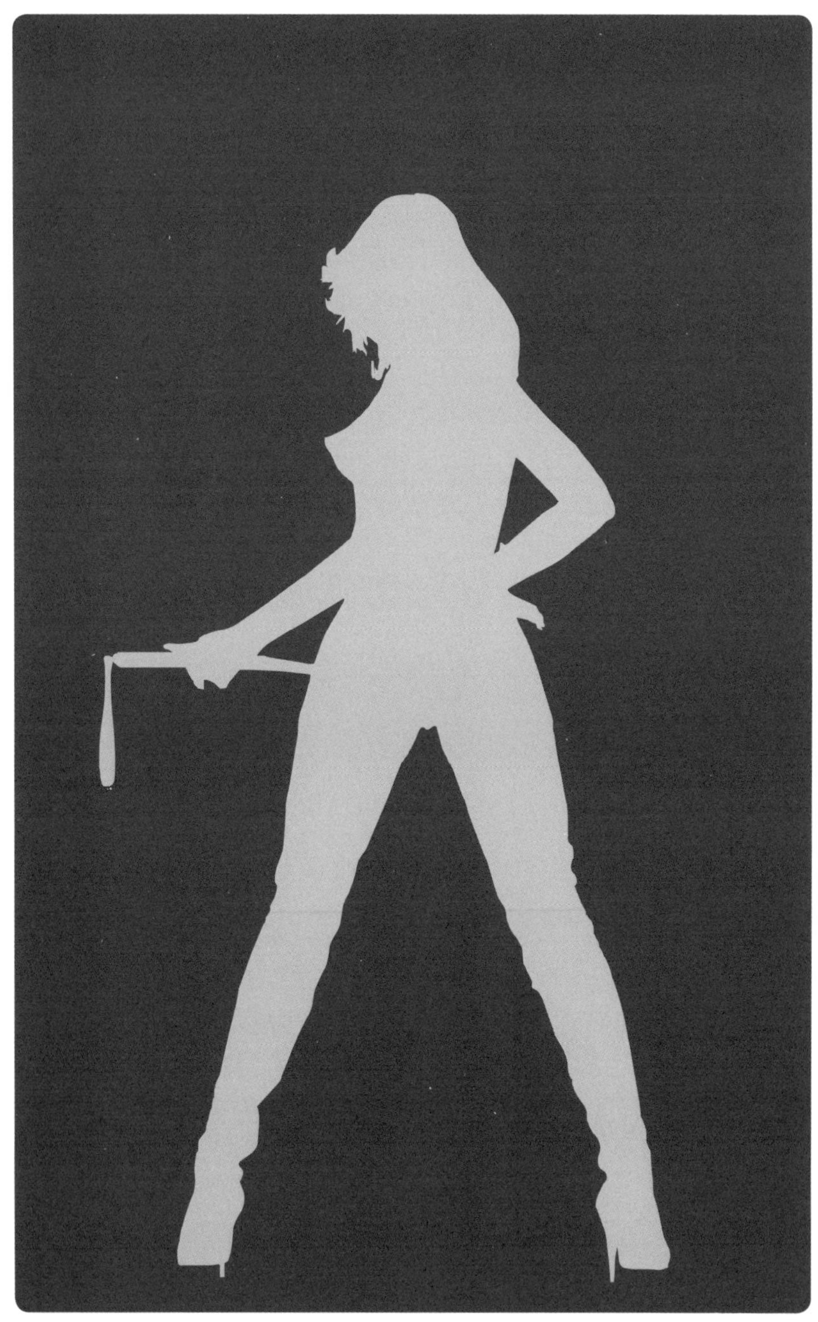

3
Power Games

POWER AND SEX ARE INEXTRICABLY ENTWINED. THEY DO SAY THAT POWER IS THE GREATEST APHRODISIAC – IT MUST BE, BECAUSE OTHERWISE HOW COULD YOU EXPLAIN THE APPARENTLY IRRESISTIBLE CHARM OF SOME OF THE WORLD'S RICHEST, MOST COMMANDING BUT UGLIEST MEN?

When we have difficulties in our own love lives, often it's because we feel powerless. We don't feel able to say what we want to be in control of, whether our own needs or what happens between us and a partner. Setting up a situation where you agree one of you is absolutely in control can be a great liberator. It makes the one in charge feel competent and strong. It can also be quite a relief to the other one. You may only feel bad about not having a say when you think you should be making choices. When you agree to be told and led, you can relax and not worry, handing the reins over to the other person. That's also the reason why it works particularly well when you reverse the normal order of things, letting the one who's usually in charge in your relationship take a back seat and handing control to the one who is usually looked after.

Set the scene by arranging a corner of a room like an office, with a desk and chair, a desk lamp if you have one, papers and pens. Dress in "business" clothes – a suit for him or dark trousers and a shirt and tie, sober skirt and blouse for her. But underneath, she should be wearing stockings rather than tights and a sexy bra. She should use a strap as a belt. Imagine you're at the end of a busy day. You have a deadline coming up and an important project that has to be completed or the company is in trouble. She's the boss, a powerful lady who has high standards and never lets a mistake go by without soundly reprimanding the person who made it. He's her assistant, in awe of her, and he's made an error. He's been sitting there, nervous and on edge, hoping against hope she'll not have noticed it or will have decided to correct it herself, for speed. Some hope!

Start the action by having him sitting at his desk. She should then come in, and throw a sheaf of papers over him. Alternatively, if you have a mobile phone, she could ring him at his desk and order him into her inner sanctum. Or, she could set this up by ringing him earlier in the day, at his real place of work, to make an appointment, to tell him exactly what time he should go in to see her. Once there, she shouts the ceiling down. She's furious, and she's going to make sure he knows exactly how annoyed she is, and make him pay for putting her out. You could agree your own dialogue earlier, or use this: "For heaven's sake, look at this work – it's a mess. What did you think you were doing? I've a good mind to get rid of you." "Look, I'm really sorry. I'm sure I can fix it, just give me some time." He should plead, abjectly, for her understanding and forgiveness, but she remains unmoved and isn't going to forgive easily. "We don't have the time, you idiot. You're such an incompetent fool I've done it myself. In fact, the job's finished and done with, thanks to me and no thanks to you. So now everyone else has gone home and if you don't want the sack, you'll have to take your punishment." She strips off his tie and uses it to tie him to his chair. Hiking up her skirt to show her stocking tops, she then puts a hand down his trousers and brings him to attention. What happens next is designed to underline just how much in control she is, and how powerless and under her thumb he has become. With one hand stroking him and the other exposing her breasts to tease him, she laughs at him. "I bet you'd like to have a taste of these, wouldn't you? But you're far too incompetent to know what to do, you'll just have to let me show you how to do it!" He can beg for release and for the chance to show how good he can be, but she just keeps on teasing him. She unzips his trousers, slips off her underwear and mounts him, all the while telling him that if he doesn't do a better job of staying erect than he did of the paperwork, he'll be really sorry. The boss may agree to untie him – but only so she can order her underling to go on his knees to kiss her feet, to perform oral sex, to grovel for her attention. He has to obey, because she's in charge.

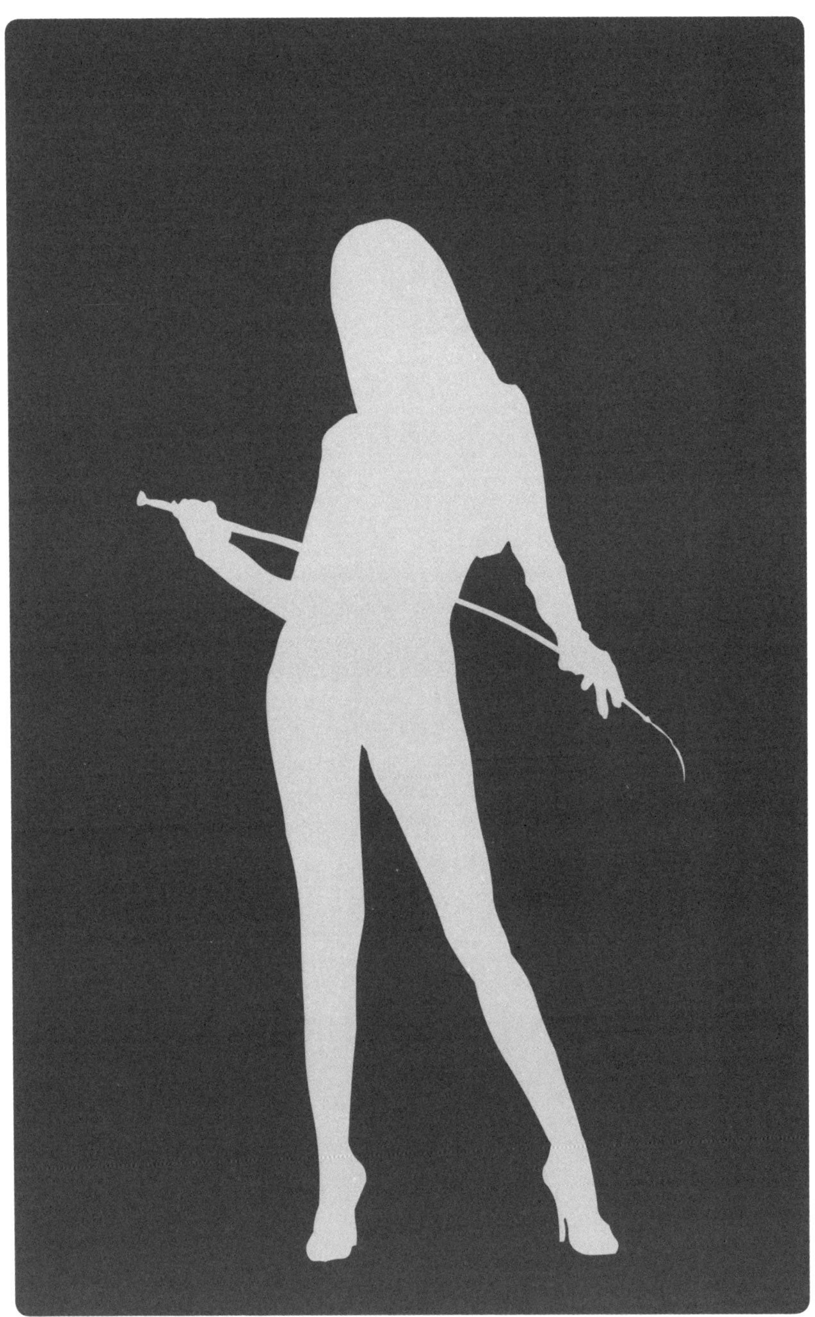

"4"
All Tied Up

BONDAGE IS ALL ABOUT GIVING YOURSELF PERMISSION TO ACT IN WAYS YOU'VE ALWAYS FELT WERE SINFUL. MOST OF US WOULD LOVE TO HAVE SEX WITH WILD ABANDON, TO REVEL AND ROLL IN DELICIOUS NAUGHTINESS.

What often holds us back is the fear that we'll get told off or feel bad. In the back of our minds sits nanny or a parent saying, "This is disgusting, you shouldn't be doing it. How dare you, you wicked child!" But when someone ties us up and forces us to get aroused, to have sex, to satisfy them, it's not our fault. Being tied up relieves us of all responsibility for what ensues, and that's a wonderfully liberating feeling. We can be as wicked and wanton as we like, all the while protesting, "But I can't help it. Look, I'm being made to do this!" The more you struggle against your bonds, the more you can protest it was none of your choice and none of your fault – and the more you can enjoy it. Introducing a bit of punishment into the game makes it even more comforting. As you are spanked or beaten, you can soothe any lingering feelings of guilt for enjoying what's happening. It's as if you say, "Yes, I know I'm being depraved, but look, I'm being punished so I don't have to feel bad about it."

Set the scene by dressing for your parts. If she is to be Miss Whiplash, she needs Lycra or PVC clothing in the form of a tight, revealing bodysuit. She can wear straps and chains and should have stiletto heels and carry a whip or cane. If he is to be Mr. Correction, he could be in a leather harness and brief leather or Lycra shorts. The aim is for the dominator to look as fearsome and hard as possible. The victim should be dressed in ordinary, light street clothes, but have on a thong so their buttocks are on show when they strip down. The effect you want is for the victim to feel vulnerable and exposed, so any clothing that might give them protection or comfort is out.

Arrange your room to resemble a dungeon. You should have dark drapes and plenty of large candles to give a dim, flickering light. Have an assortment of places where the victim can be tied up – then get into character. The victim is shivering with anticipation, scared yet excited. The dominator has no fears and no concerns but is in charge – absolutely. They should be waiting, whip in hand and foot tapping.

Start the action by having the victim knock on the door, nervously. They are answered by a fearsome creature, who snaps, "Hello, worm. Come in, strip off, don't give me any lip and do as you're told!" The dominator is sure and in control. They know what the victim needs and are about to give it to them. The victim is led into the dungeon and made to strip down to a thong. As they take off each piece of clothing, the dominator prods them with the whip and sneers. "What a miserable body, you really do need some correction, don't you?" "Yes, Boss, whatever you say, Boss." The victim is blindfolded and tied up and then the dominator throws the dice, and interpreting the instruction as they see fit, the dominator then uses either feather or whip together, or one after the other, to tickle and spank. "Don't get aroused or you'll be sorry," or "Don't you dare come without my permission," or "Come on, let's have a bit of action here," they'll demand as they arouse but delay the victim's climax. The dominator will take their own satisfaction from the victim's cringing body but the victim can only submit. The victim is allowed to come only when the dominator says they may.

TOP TIP

Pleasure and pain are surprisingly close. When you become sexually aroused, your nipples, genitals and lips become engorged with blood, swell and heat up. When you smack an arm, a leg or buttock, it smarts and also becomes hot and sensitive. Make your buttocks tingle from a spanking and your mind will often become confused, telling your body that the sensation is actually arousal. Plenty of people find it highly stirring to have small, measured and controlled amounts of pain inflicted during sex play by their partners.

Doctor & Nurse

MOST OF US SUFFER FROM THE SNEAKING
FEELING THAT ENJOYING SEX IS NOT ALLOWED.
OUR FIRST, EARLY EXPLORATIONS OF OUR
BODIES WERE PROBABLY MET WITH SLAPPED
HANDS AND A TELLING OFF.

We knew that authority, in the form of our parents, didn't approve, which is why Doctors and Nurses is such a popular game for children.

It's such a good excuse to let those hands roam free, as we find out what feels good and which parts of the body differ from little girls to little boys. Most young people play Doctors and Nurses at some time, as a cover for early sexual curiosity. We know that medical personnel are only doing their job when they have you on the couch, undressed and open to their examination. If you were a doctor or a nurse, it would be perfectly OK for you to have your hands all over the unclothed body of your patients. It's also OK for a patient to be seen by a doctor, even when they may feel too shy to be seen by anyone else. This is why Doctor and Nurse is an excellent game for big boys and girls,

too. It allows you the perfect opportunity to twiddle this and tweak that, to stroke and knead with impunity. After all, the doctor is only doing his or her job, examining the patients to make it all better. And the patient is only doing the proper thing in turn, by accepting the doctor's administrations, and helping out by indicating where it hurts and where it does not.

Set the scene by arranging your chosen room as an examination cubicle. Have a single divan, sofa or table covered with a towel or sheet, to stand in for the examination couch. Lay out a tray of instruments – a container of lubricating cream, jelly or oil, surgical gloves and a vibrator. Get your uniforms prepared. You're to be doctor and nurse in a busy hospital. Don't forget that there are male nurses and female doctors, so you can try taking your

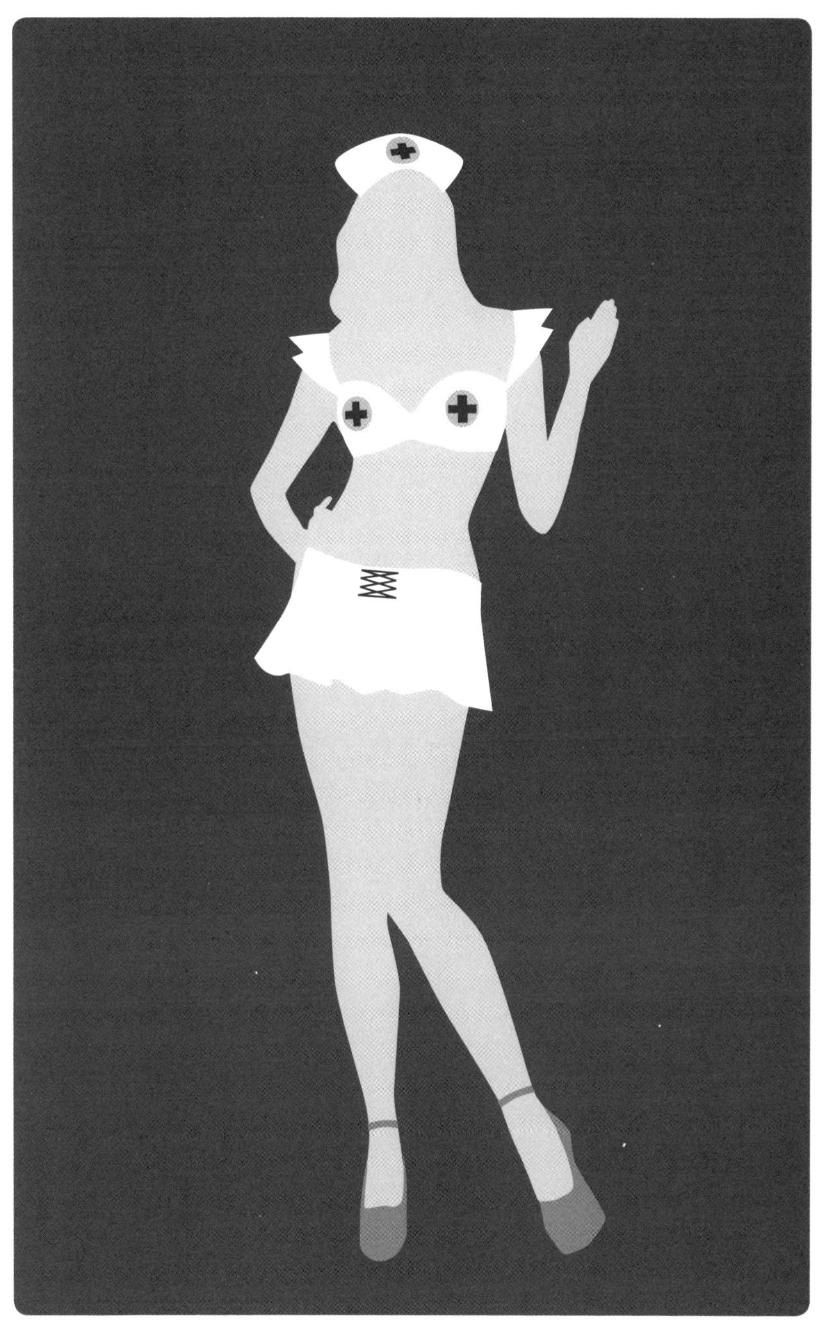

turns in either role. One of you is a doctor in scrubs worn in operating theatres or a doctor's coat – a green or blue loose cotton jacket and tie-waist trousers. The other is in a plain shirt and skirt/trousers for the nurses uniform or also in "scrubs." The doctor is the one in authority, someone the nurse admires and will listen to. Anything a doctor suggests must be for their own good, so the nurse is going to take heed and follow the doctor's suggestions.

Start the action by imagining it's been a hard night. As the nurse passes the doctor's room, the doctor calls out, "You look worn out, nurse. Got a headache?" "Yes, doctor, I can't seem to get rid of it." "Well, I know a cure for that, nurse. Hop up on the couch and I'll give you a neck message." Nurse lies down and the doctor says, "I'm really good at relieving tension this way, nurse. Just tell me if this feels good." The doctor then proceeds to stroke and massage the nurse's neck and back, unbuttoning and pushing down or pulling up the nurse's uniform to reach the neck. A grateful nurse can say, "Oh, doctor, you do have healing hands." To keep in role, both of you should only address each other as "doctor" or "nurse." As the doctor strokes the nurse's neck and back, one hand strays to other parts of the body. "You're really tense, nurse. You should have a proper massage, you know. I read in an old medical book that this can help." (The Victorians believed that tension resulted from what they called congestion. Congestion, they thought, was relieved when the sexual organs were massaged to the point where the patient became suddenly relaxed and relieved.)

The doctor should produce a vibrator and, after gently unbuttoning the nurse's uniform, proceed to give medically prescribed treatment. The doctor can press the buzzing vibrator to the nurse's nipples, down the belly and around the genitals, asking, "Does this feel better?" Nurse can say, "Oh yes, doctor. But it really does feel tense here… and here… and here," showing the doctor where it hurts and where best to give help. The doctor can use a feather in the absence of a vibrator, or both.

TOP TIP

You can really make that hospital atmosphere come alive with a visit to your pharmacy. Buy some surgical gloves and snap them on, not forgetting to wash your hands thoroughly beforehand to get in the mood. And get some hospital disinfectant to splash on the towel or sheet for a really authentic smell that will transport you to your local emergency room.

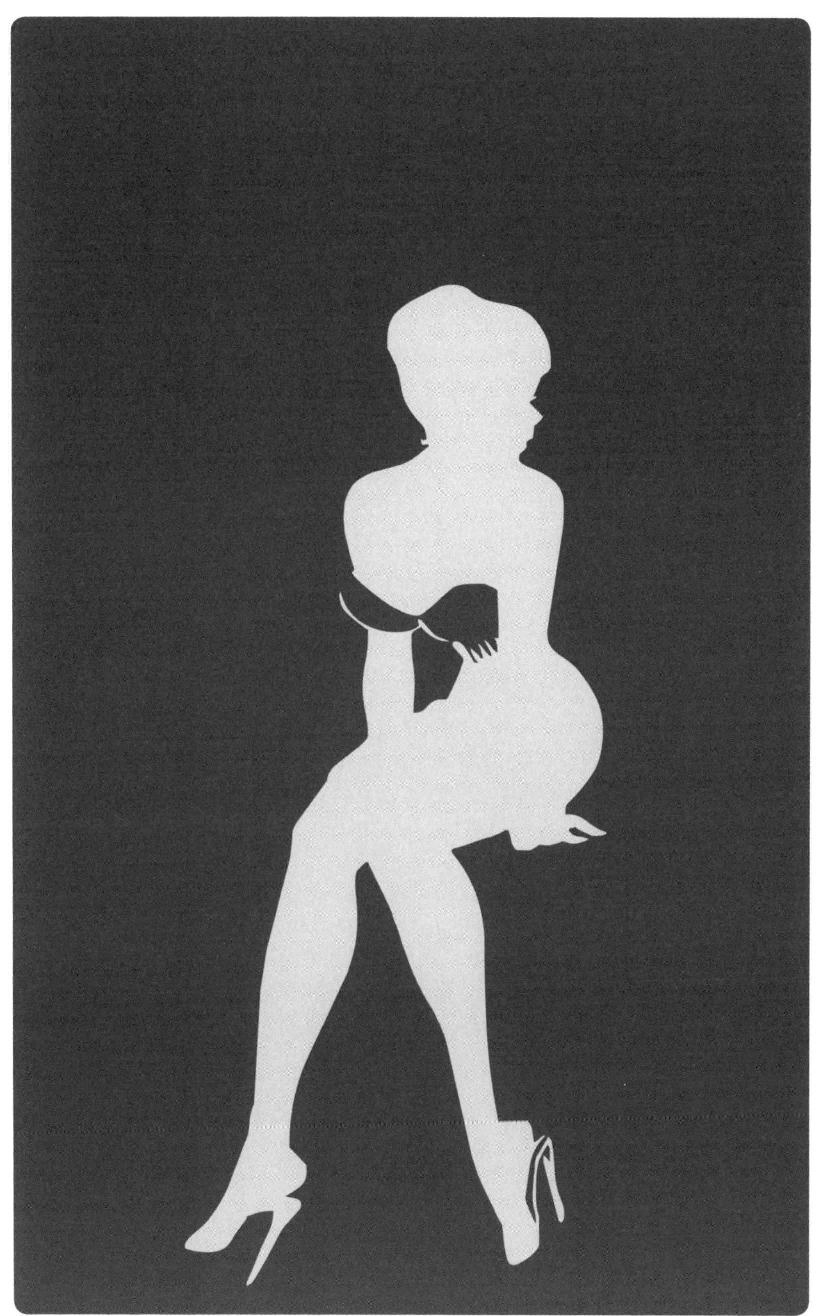

"6"
Stranger in the Night

WHEN YOU'RE LIVING TOGETHER IN A SETTLED RELATIONSHIP, MAKING SPECIAL TIME TO BE ALONE AS A COUPLE CAN OFTEN GO BY THE BOARD. RELATIONSHIPS CAN ALSO VERY EASILY GET INTO A RUT.

When you were in your early days together, your sex lives were all adventure. Every encounter was thrilling as you discovered new things about each other and yourselves. Months or years on, it's all a bit stale and the excitement has gone. You hardly ever go out and when you do, it is to do the same old things, in the same old fashion. You might be tempted to recapture the heady delight of a fresh encounter by flirting with a friend, neighbour, work-mate or even a stranger, and possibly of having an affair. Stranger in the Night allows you to experience all this, in safety, with your own lover.

Set the scene by arranging a table in the kitchen or living room to resemble a bar or café, with cups of coffee or drinks. Put on a coat if it's winter but don't wear anything underneath except your underwear, and make sure it's your briefest and sexiest. If it's summer, dress in outdoor clothes but with nothing on underneath. He should be carrying a newspaper. You're both single, on your own and simply enjoying a quiet moment in a busy life.

Start the action with one of you sitting down and having a cup of coffee or a drink at the café or bar table. Of course, if you really want to go the whole hog, play this for real. Make a date to meet up somewhere new, where you aren't known. Pretend you don't know each other. So whether you're at home or out, once one of you is settled, the other should come up and ask to share the table. Take a few moments to give each other a "once over" secretly. What do you find attractive? What particular part of their body would you like to touch? What would you like to do to and with them? When you've looked your fill, strike up a conversation. "Do

you come here often? What do you do with
your free time? Do you have a partner or are
you available?" Let the conversation become
more intimate. "What sort of person do you
find yourself falling for? What sort of sex do
you like?" As the chat gets hotter, she can let
her coat fall open to show she is just in her
underwear, or pull up her skirt to show she
isn't wearing any. He can casually remark
that he's wearing a thong. Under the table
and under the cover of coats or a newspaper,
both of you should let a hand sneak out to
touch, fondle and explore the other's body.
You can go as far as you like if the "café" is a
pretence. How far you go if you're in a real
bar is up to you, the lighting and the bar's
other customers.

TOP TIP

*Doing this for real can give you extra
kicks, but do be careful. Don't do
anything intimate when or where you
could be seen or discovered and cause
offence or discomfort to others. Not only
is it bad manners, it's also illegal and
can get you into considerable trouble.
The best compromise is to pick each
other up in public but continue
other activities once you get to
somewhere private.*

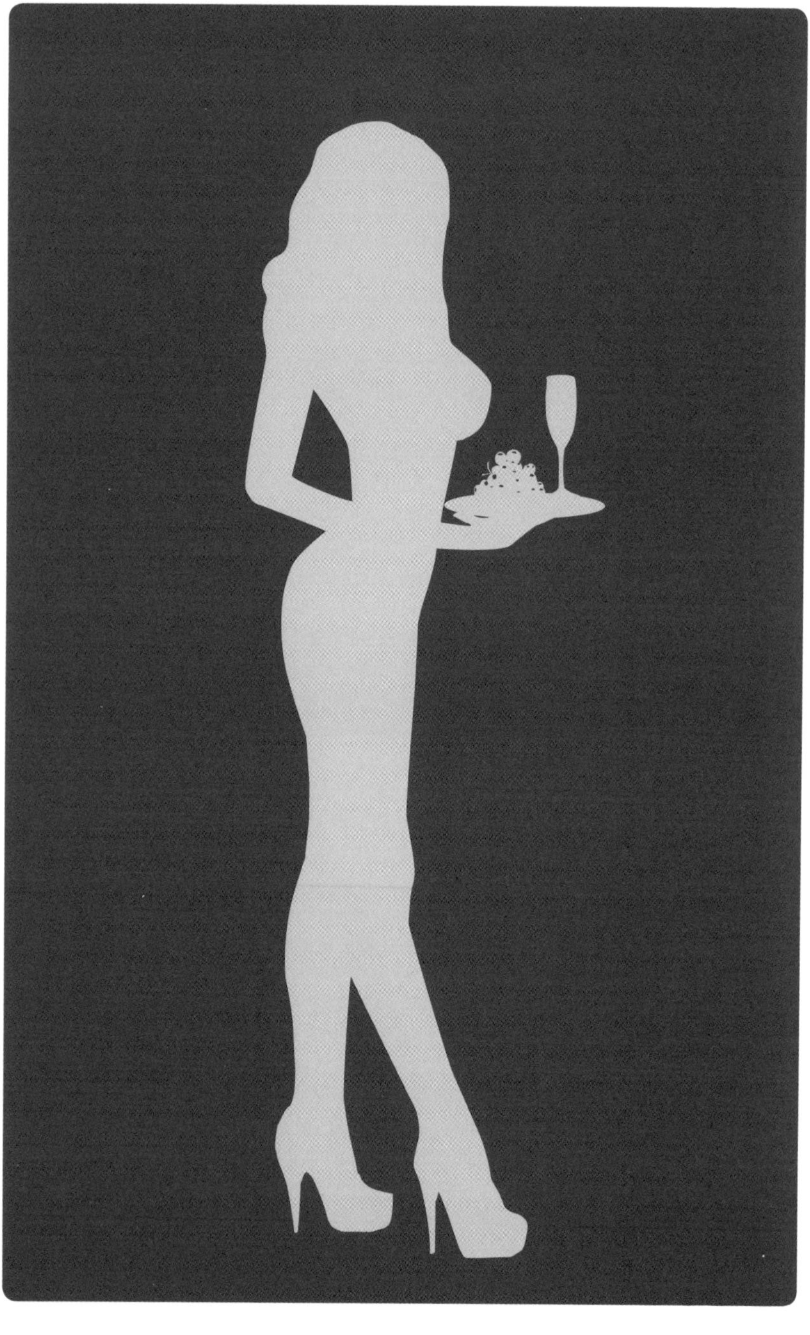

7
Feast of Love

FOOD AND DRINK OFTEN ENHANCE SEX, BUT
A CANDLELIT DINNER ISN'T ONLY ROMANTIC
BECAUSE YOUR COMPANION LOOKS ENTICING
IN THE FLICKERING LIGHT.

It's because, as you nibble, lick and slurp your food, both of you are sending the message that you would like to do the same to various parts of your lover's body. And some foods are inextricably linked to sex.

We believe that many edibles have the power to affect our sex lives, by increasing our sexual desire or sexual capabilities. Long, penis-shaped foods such as bananas or asparagus, and substances such as powdered rhino horn, are reputed to give men vigorous erections and make them potent. Figs, which look like the inside of a vulva, and oysters, which have an intimate feminine odour, are supposed to put both sexes in the mood for love. Hot, spicy foods such as curry and chilli are reputed to raise the temperature, put us in mind of aromatic and sweaty encounters and to heat the sexual organs directly. And, of course, drinks such as champagne have always had a sexy reputation. The bubbles get up your nose, loosen your inhibitions and put you in the mood for other frothy explosions.

Set the scene for Feast of Love with a shopping trip, stocking up with as much of the special foods and drink as you can afford. Prepare your room as a harem or an "Arabian Nights" palace. Turn the lights low, and have the room lit by candles on every surface. Pile the cushions or pillows on the bed or floor, and spread plates, bowls, bottles and glasses full of food and drink all around you. Dress yourselves in Eastern-style clothing, such as kaftans or kimonos, or tie and drape sarongs of silk-type scarves over yourself. Start the action by imagining you're both sensualists, about to embark on an evening of pleasure, with all the time in the world. Anything that feels good and pleases your partner too is allowed. You're going to work your way through the food and drink and devour each other as well. You know you're good enough to eat, and your partner is about to prove it. Slowly and seductively, feed titbits to each other. Pick up a peach, a fig, a spear of asparagus or bar of crumbly chocolate, as is appropriate, and lick, suck and nibble, saying, "This reminds me of you – is this what you'd like me to do to you?" Dribble spoonfuls of wine, cream or ice cream on each other and lick it off. Swallow mouthfuls of curry or warm chocolate, of figs or asparagus, and imagine them going straight to your nipples and clitoris, or to your penis. Just visualize the warmth and taste, shape and feel affecting you, making you swollen and hot, ready for love. Eat sparingly and slowly so you don't get over full and bloated, but taste and devour a bit of everything and share small mouthfuls with your partner, to make the point and get the idea. Revel in contrasts. You can switch from hot to cold by taking a mouthful of ice or ice cream and then tonguing or sucking a part of your partner's body – earlobe or nipple, penis or clitoris. Having chilled

and stimulated them, take a mouthful of something warm and repeat the exercise. Go from something crunchy and fresh to something sloppy and rich, and see how the contrasting texture compares to your partner's body. The beauty of this game is that it is, in fact, very flexible. You can surround yourself with the entire contents of a supermarket trolley. Or you can do it with just a takeaway and a can of lager, or a tub of ice cream. If you really want to go to town, you can put down a rubber sheet and pour your food all over each other and eat it off your partner's body.

TOP TIP

Having strenuous sex on a full stomach isn't a recipe for love. Feast of Love is best done with tiny treats, luxurious nibbles and tasty titbits. Graze your way through a sumptuous spread, but make sure you actually eat small amounts, over a period of time.

"8"
Three's Not a Crowd

The temptation to make love to – or be made love to by – more than just your own partner at a time comes from a wish to have your ego massaged as well as your body.

If you can cope with more than one lover, it suggests that your sexual abilities are extreme. You can believe that your sexual desires are so great that it needs more than one person to satisfy you. It also appeals to the exhibitionist in us, the thought of having someone else watching as we make love to a third person, approving of us and admiring our moves. Whatever, thinking that there are extra bodies in the bed with you can really put a kick into the proceedings. Carrying it out for real, however, can cause problems. You have the worry of sexual infections, and also the fear of competition and emotional entanglements. The last thing you want is for your partner to decide someone else does it better for them, or for you to fall for a person other than your partner, and have to deal with the problems this creates. Take it from me, this is one of those fantasies – and there are plenty – that is more attractive in the imagination than in reality. Playing Three's Not a Crowd allows you to experience the thrill with none of the drawbacks.

Prepare the scene by placing one or more large mirrors around you where you are going to make love – in the bedroom, bathroom or living room. You can place one upright against a wall and/or prop one up along the side of the bed, so it will reflect you as you lie down. If you don't have any suitable mirrors, create the illusion of other people by using a blindfold and suggestion. Turn the lights down low, perhaps illuminating the room just with candles or the light from a door left ajar. Have a blindfold on hand as you go to your partner.

Start the action by putting on some music. Choose a smoochy, sexy number, and one that is not just instrumental. Make sure

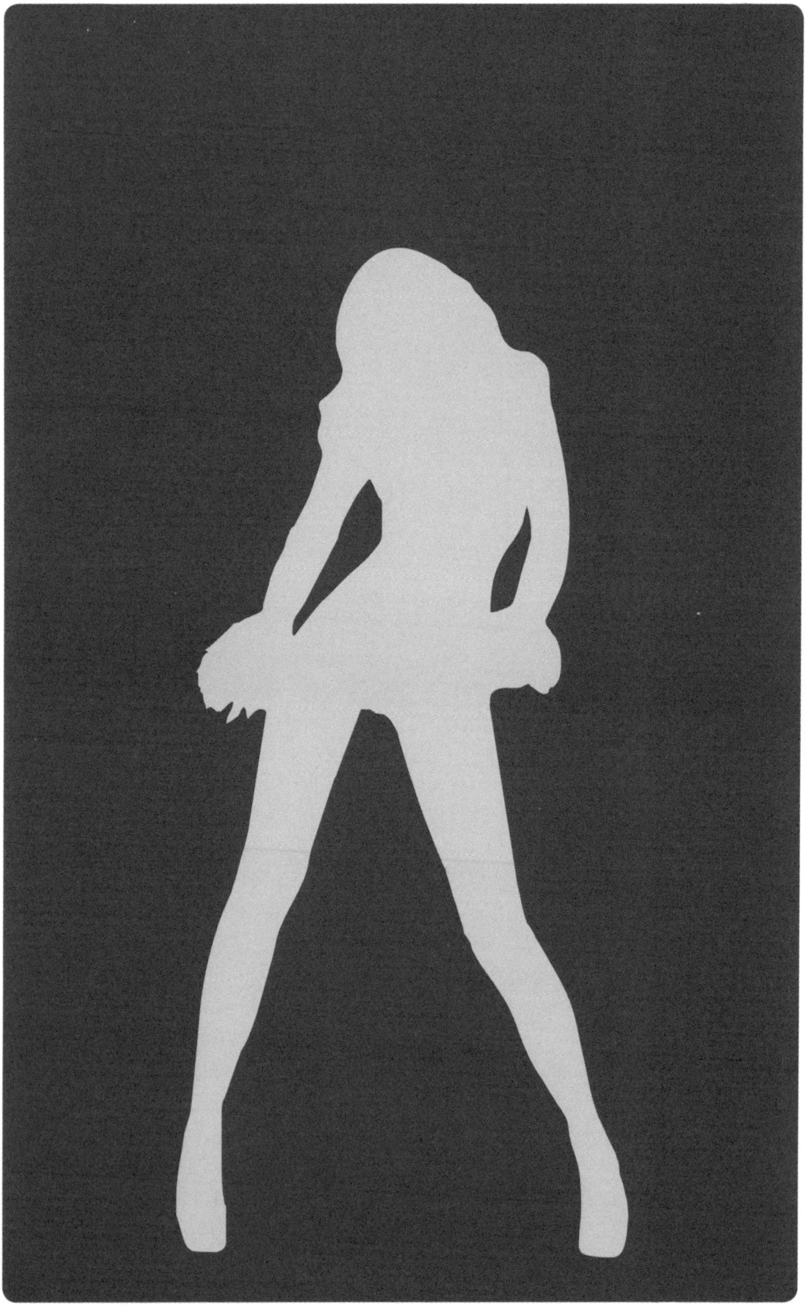

there are voices apart from your own to be heard. Then begin to cosy up to your partner, saying, "You know we've been talking about those friends of ours who like to swing? Let's go upstairs, because I think they're planning to join us tonight." Blindfold your partner and lead them up to the dimly lit bedroom. Start seducing your partner, kissing and caressing them and undressing them, pressed up against the mirror if you have one. When both of you are fully aroused, say, "Whose hands are these? Are they mine or are they John's or Jane's?" If you've a mirror, slide the blindfold off and allow your partner to see reflections, in the half-light. If not, keep the blindfold fully or partly on. You could throw the dice, to choose which action and to which part of the body you and your "friends" should be paying special attention. Keep up a running commentary about what the other people in the room are doing to your partner, and to each other and to you. "He's touching you on your breast. Now she's holding me. That's his hand between your legs. Can you hear her coming?" Use a vibrator, a feather or a silk glove to make sure that both of you feel different textures and temperatures in the touches you are experiencing all over your bodies.

TOP TIP

Ever had someone sneak up behind you, cover your eyes and cry, "Guess who?" You can usually tell if it's your partner by their smell, whether you realize it or not. You know the soap, the toothpaste and cologne they normally use. But you can also identify that subtle odour that is their own body smell, and which is highly sexy to your nose. This can make it hard to establish the illusion of it being someone else. To make you feel that it isn't only the two of you in the bedroom, splash the pillow beforehand with a perfume or aftershave that neither of you wears.

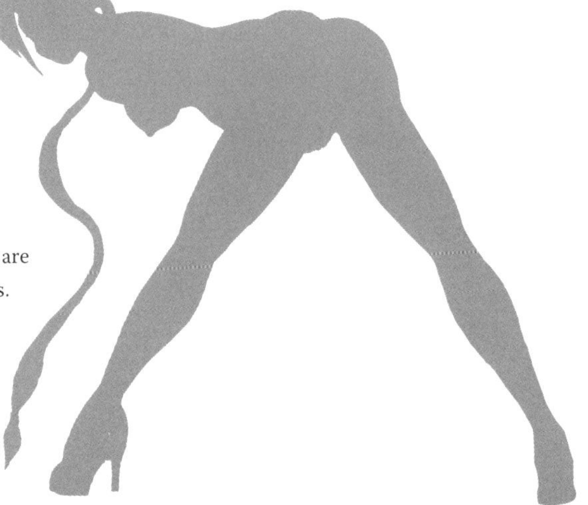

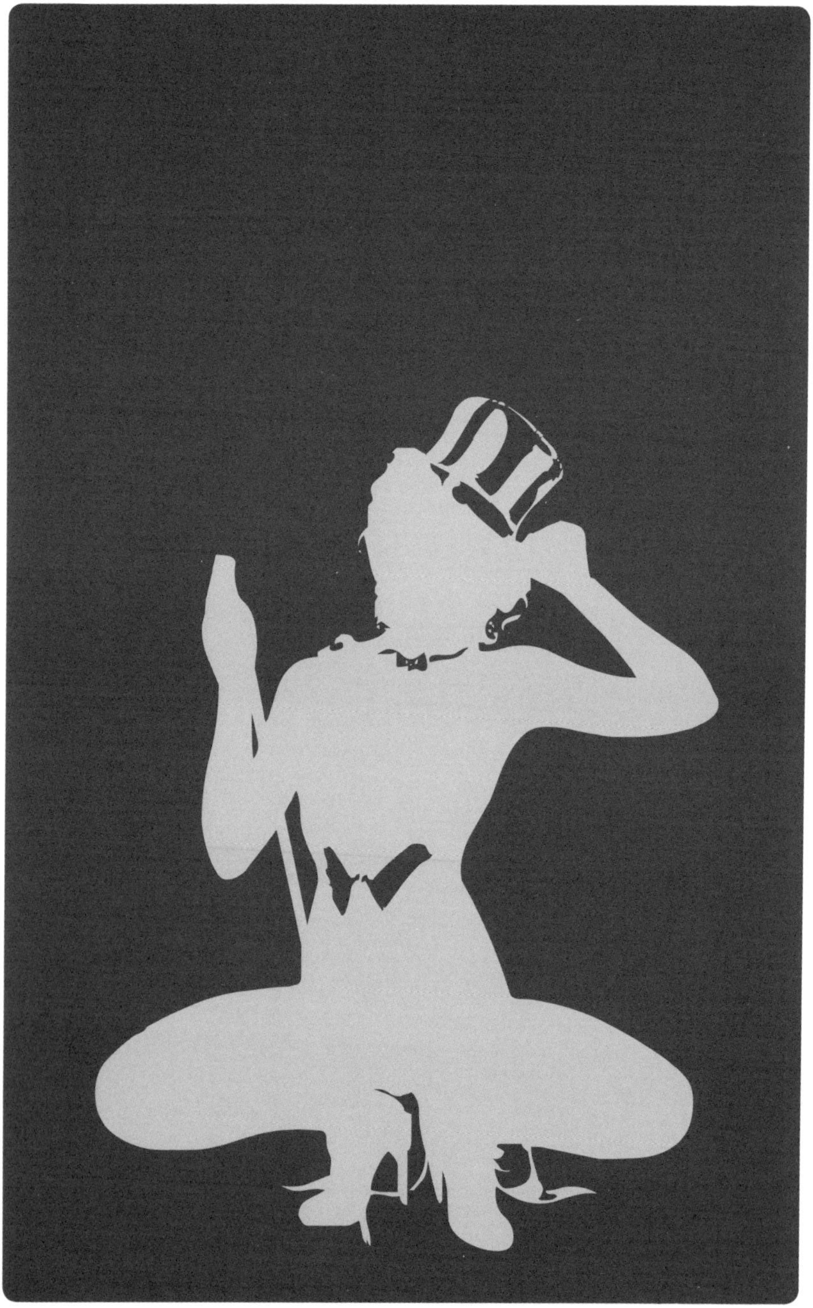

9
You're the Act

WE ALL FEEL A BIT UNSURE OF OUR SKILLS IN BED. WE'D LOVE TO THINK THAT WE'RE SEXUAL EXPERTS, BUT MOST US FEAR THAT WE'RE ACTUALLY SEXUALLY INEPT, WHICH IS WHY IMAGINING YOU'RE THE HEADLINE ACT IN A SEX SHOW IS A VERY POPULAR SEXUAL FANTASY.

Picture yourself in front of an eager, admiring, applauding audience. By imagining your fans urging you on to new heights as you demonstrate your skills in the art of sex, you can give yourselves more than a thrill. It can also help you both feel more confident in yourselves and be more confident in the way you please each other. As you think about people watching, envying and wanting to copy you, you can start accepting that perhaps what you're doing and the way you're doing it is worth some praise.

Arrange the scene by making a stage set in your bedroom or living room. You can use a rug to outline the limits of a small stage, or use your own bed as the set. Dim the lights, leaving one light – the spotlight – shining on the central area. Pick a soundtrack with a pounding beat and appropriate lyrics that get you going – and make sure you have at least an hour of music to work to. Have a container of oil or cream within reach, then prepare yourselves. Use glamour make-up to give yourselves a stage sparkle. Dust glitter make-up on breasts, backsides and genitals. Dress in thongs and clothes that you can shrug out of and remove easily. You'll both be feeling the butterflies that any performer gets before a show, but also the quiet confidence of true professionals. You're so good at this, you know you're going to get a good reception and show your audience a thing or two.

As you hear the music coming up to your big number, start the action by putting the final touches to your make-up and costumes and making your entrance. Step into the spotlight, twirl each other round with a shimmy and a shake and get down to business. Strip each other of your clothes. Take your time about it – each article should come off slowly, with a tease and a flourish. When you're down to nothing, fetch the bottle of oil or cream from the side of the stage and slowly spread it all over each other. Arouse and excite each other and, to the imagined howls and screams of your frenzied audience, make love on the stage in front of them all. Every move should be larger than life, played to the gallery. You can imagine your fans at the back of the room standing on the tables and urging you on, and your gestures should be large enough for them to be able to see exactly what you are doing to each other. After all, this is what they've paid to see. Afterward, don't forget to congratulate and praise each other, as real performers do. A few high-fives and "Nice moves!" will finish the act properly.

Of course, you can make up your own act. Boogie Nights and Disco Dancing aren't the only ways to perform a live sex act in front of an audience. Perhaps you'd like to imagine yourselves doing a Dracula, sweeping a cloak over your partner as you gnaw at their neck. Or being a Gladiator, knocking holes out of each other in your Lycra and helmets before getting down on the mats. Or one of you can do a solo performance, pleasuring themselves for the audience of one. Or you can start the act with one of you in the audience, being invited up to strut your stuff with the professional performer. It's your script so get writing!

Make a recording of a stage show, one that has plenty of audience participation in the form of whoops, claps and shouted comments. Play it as you perform You're the Act and try to pace your performance to the audience reaction.

10
Paying for It

When you are paid, you can feel that this "sex money" confirms that you're special. Similarly, imagining that your "mark" is prepared to give you cash for the privilege of having sex with you says that you and what you're offering is so good that it deserves such recognition and reward.

When you are the one doing the paying, there is a different advantage. The customer is always right. If you're buying it, you can be totally self-seeking. You don't have to think about the other person's needs or pleasures but can concentrate on satisfying yourself and yourself only. You can also specify exactly what it is you want, without having to be shy, embarrassed or unselfish. This is why so many men use prostitutes in real life – the fact that they can get what they want and not have to bother about wooing and courting or thinking about the other person's needs. The other reason is that paid sex is felt to be "dirty" sex. And, often, there's nothing quite as thrilling and stimulating as being very naughty indeed. It's like sloshing around making mud pies. There's plenty of fun in the sheer sensuality of feeling it squish between your fingers, but even more enjoyment to be had from the knowledge that Mother has told you not to. Imagining you're involved in the contract of buying and selling can make your sexual encounter seem sleazy and bad. And while that's not a recipe for happy sex in real life, it can be a definite turn-on in fantasy time.

Set the scene by dressing the part. The one who is to act as the sex worker should put on tight, revealing and cheap clothes. She can dress like a tart, in a very short skirt or Lycra leggings and cropped top with heavy make-up. If he's to be the rent boy, tight jeans or cut-offs, a T-shirt with cap sleeves or a shirt open to the waist will do. We tend to assume that all straight sex workers are women, and all clients are

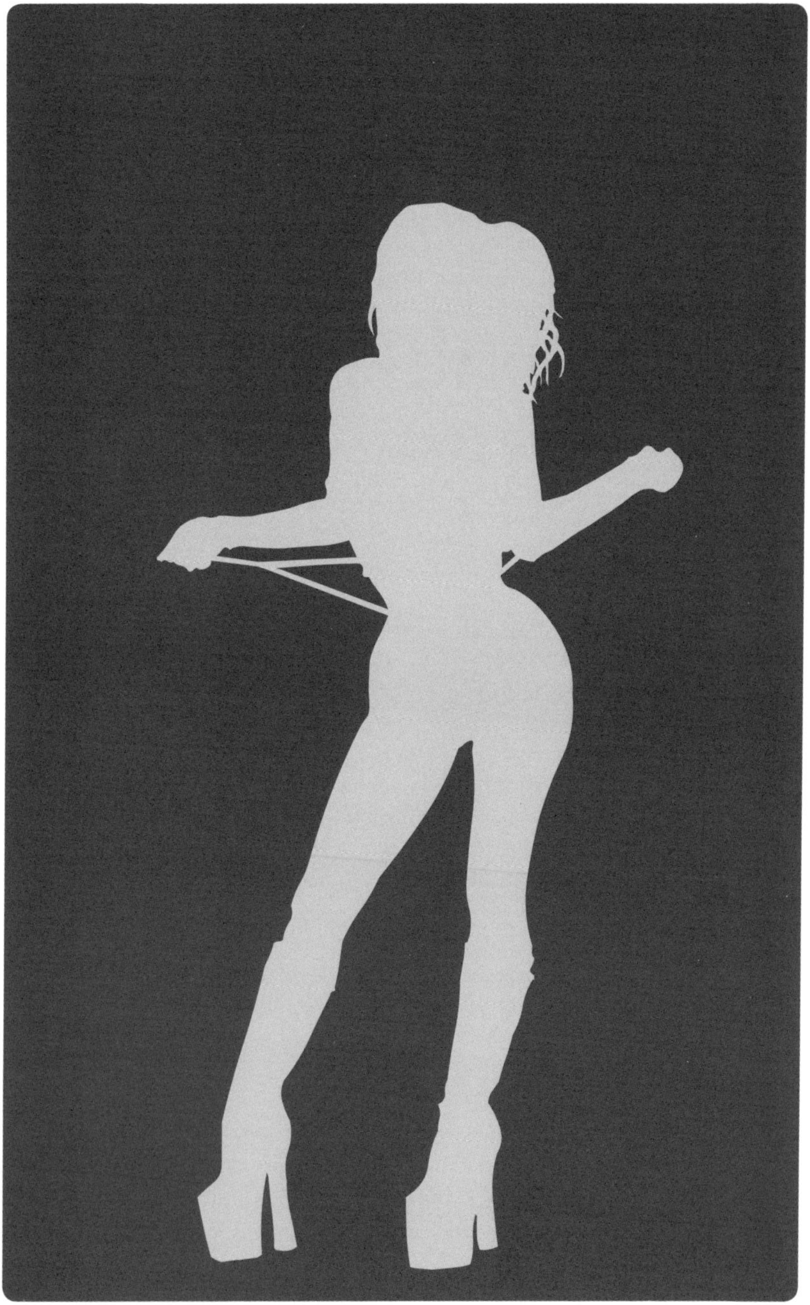

men. That isn't actually true, and certainly shouldn't cramp your style. If she's going to get a kick out of being good enough to be paid to do it, so is he.

Both of you are likely to be a bit nervous. The sex worker is world-weary and cynical, having seen it all before. Nothing a client asks for can shock or surprise. Start the action by having the buyer, feeling excited and determined to get what they want, approach the sex worker and ask, "Are you available?" to which the response might be, "Depends. What are you looking for?" The buyer can then say exactly what they'd like. It might be a quickie, for sex standing up in an alleyway; a hand-job, for masturbation; an oral, for oral sex; or round the world, for everything – oral, anal and straight sex. You could specify that you want the sex worker to do all the work, making you come while you lie there being serviced; or you can insist that you want to take your pleasure from them as they stand or lie there, not moving. Or, you can ask that the sex is like making love – but they do have to touch and caress you as and when you tell them to. "That'll cost you," the sex worker can say, and they should name a price. Or they may object to what's asked for and name another similar but easier sex act. The sex worker may also, for authenticity, demand, "And you'll have to wear a condom," and then be prepared to haggle if the client says, "I'll pay you double

to let me ride bareback." When they finally agree and the buyer hands over the cash, the sex worker leads the way up to the bedroom. Once the price is paid, the worker has to do what the customer says, as long as it is what they have asked and paid for.

TOP TIP

To introduce an extra edge to the negotiations, use real money. The sex worker gets to keep the cash and buy themselves a treat with it.

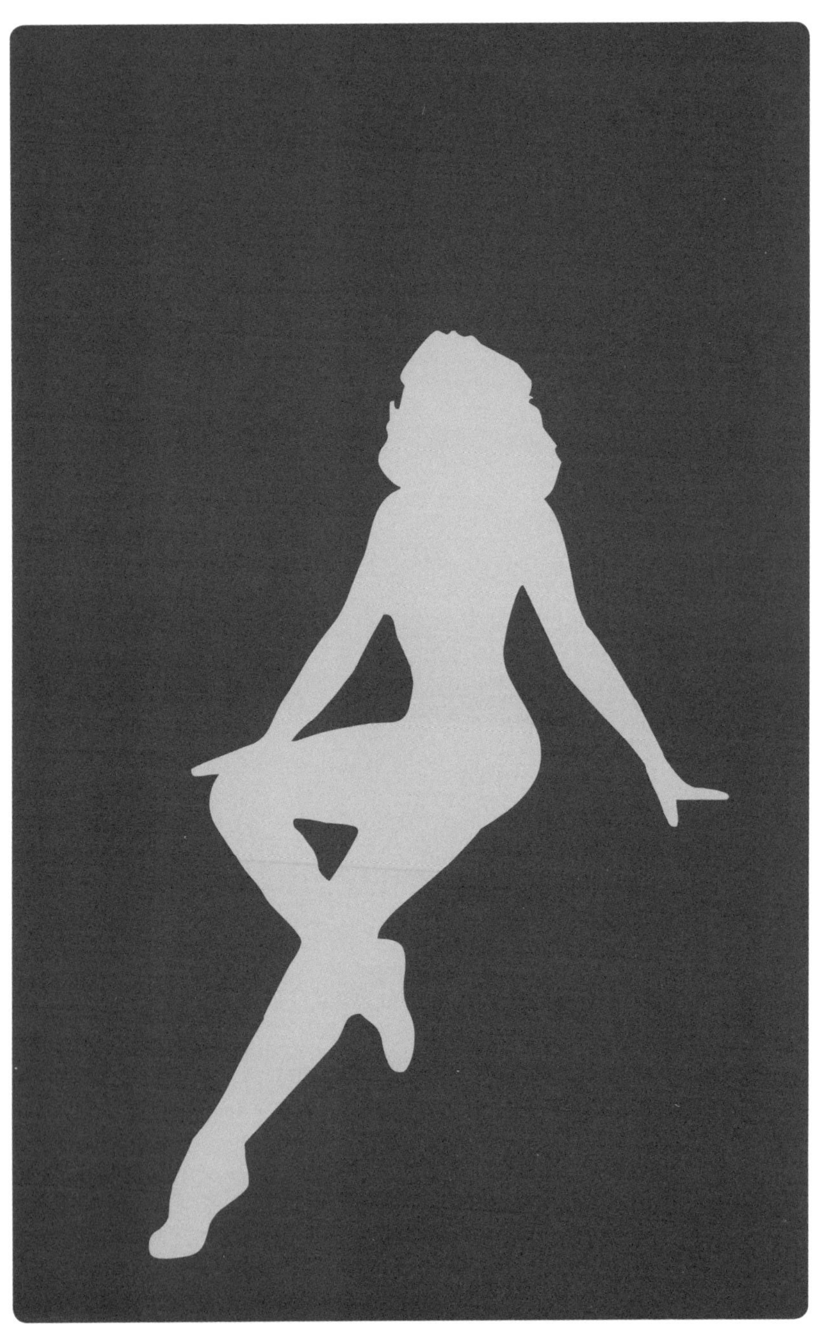

Quick One

HAVING SLOW, CONSIDERED, LOVING SEX WITH FULL FOREPLAY AND A LONG AFTERGLOW CAN BE BOTH SEXUALLY SATISFYING AND A GREAT WAY OF SHOWING YOUR FEELINGS. BUT THERE ARE TIMES WHEN A "WHAM, BAM, THANK YOU, SAM" APPROACH FITS THE BILL EVEN BETTER.

Fast and furious spur-of-the-moment sex has just as much of a loving message to pass to your partner. It tells them that you're so overcome with passion that you must, simply MUST, have them there and then. It tells them that their attraction and your feelings for them are so strong that you are prepared to risk anything to slake your immediate thirst for their body. And quickie sex, while being a bit of a cheat if that's the only sort you have, can be intensely arousing in certain situations. You'll be sure to find that the rush of adrenaline that the fear of discovery or interruption provokes, along with your insistence that you can't wait, will aid arousal and orgasm. Quickie sex is also another way to return to first base. It's in the first few months of a relationship that we experience our fiercest, most intense feelings. That goes

for the emotional link between us, as the pangs of love are at their strongest, but it's also noticeable in bed. Our sexual responses are probably at their most extreme at this time. When our relationship becomes more settled and stable, and probably more loving, the downside is that everything seems to be a bit short-lived and colourless. Quickie sex puts you back in the frame. You're doing it passionately, suddenly, spontaneously. But the feelings also follow, to suit the action. You are likely to find yourself breathless again, and not just because you're in a hurry but because your partner and your feelings for them take your breath away once more.

Quickie sex also keys into another popular sexual fantasy, that of having sex with a stranger. Many men and women say that one of their favourite daydreams is to imagine meeting someone, whose face they don't even see, and with them share a sudden and burning embrace and hurried sex, before going their separate ways again. Quickie sex can be particularly exciting because it is "no strings" sex. There's no foreplay, where you try to court and please your partner and make sure they're in the mood for love. If you compare leisurely, loving sex to a four-course banquet, which takes preparation and forethought, time and effort, quickie sex is the equivalent of the fast food hamburger. You take it on the run, scoff it down and dash. It's the ultimate "I'm pleasing myself and you can please yourself, too" sex, and can be amazingly exciting for that reason. Prepare yourself by making sure you're wearing "quick-release" clothes – something you can push aside to give you easy access for sex, but that you don't have to remove. A body stocking is a no-no, a thong or French knickers or nothing at all is fine. You can agree on a plan of action in advance, or one of you can surprise the other. Pick your moment carefully – just before you know friends or relatives are due to knock on the door at any moment adds an extra tingle. Or you could catch your partner while you're out, walking in the country or at the seaside, or in a bar, art gallery or car park. Suddenly, sidle up to or grab your partner and whisper in their ear that if you don't have sex with them that very moment, you'll explode. Kiss them passionately and hungrily. Push your partner up against a convenient wall or seat, and undo zips and buttons. Pull clothes up, down and aside, just enough to allow you to connect. With one eye peeled to make sure you won't be caught out, take your partner and have fast and furious sex. Once you are finished, pull yourself together and resume whatever it was you were doing before, or about to do. Carrying on as normal afterward is half the point of a Quick One. Instead of lying in each other's arms, basking in the afterglow, you smugly hug to yourselves the knowledge of what you've, secretly and daringly, just done.

TOP TIP

Use a condom and have some wet wipes on hand. That way, there's no mess or leakage, and after sex you can go straight on with whatever you were doing. As far as anyone else is concerned, nothing has happened – apart from that silly grin on your face, that is!

"12"
Position of the Night

THERE ARE SAID TO BE OVER 521 DIFFERENT POSITIONS FOR MAKING LOVE, BUT SO MANY PEOPLE NEVER GET MUCH PAST THE GOOD OLD MAN-ON-TOP MISSIONARY POSITION. IT'S A PITY, BECAUSE OTHER POSITIONS HAVE A LOT TO RECOMMEND THEM.

To make love in a way that truly satisfies both parties, you need to fulfil certain conditions. He needs to have the head of his penis gripped and stimulated. She needs to have her clitoris massaged and caressed. Both find arousal aided by having the obvious erogenous areas, such as lips, nipples and the inside of the thighs, and the less obvious ones, such as ear lobes, necks and backs, stroked. Man-on-top is probably the worst position of all to fulfil all these. His penis may get all the attention it needs but the angle is often wrong for her clitoris to be stimulated to her fulfilment. This is why so many women find intercourse curiously unsatisfying, even though masturbation hits the spot for them. If you want to find an over-abundance of exciting ways of pleasing each other, you need to be more adventurous in the ways you go at it. Try woman-on-top, or sitting face-to-face on a bed, the woman sitting on her partner's lap. Experiment with standing, face to face or with the man entering his partner from behind. Try lying side by side, her back to his front in the spoon position. In many of these positions, both partners' hands may be free to manipulate nipples, breasts, clitoris and testicles to their own and their partner's delight. But trying something new can be daunting. You may feel uneasy or confused, scared to show inexperience and not sure how you may be able to manage. Position of the Night is a good way of getting over the initial uncertainty.

Imagine yourselves to be sexual athletes, performing for your country in the World Sex Cup. You've both trained for years to get to the peak of athletic prowess and sexual skill. There are, however, new positions being devised all the time and you need to allow for a little clumsiness as you try them out. Just remember, practice makes perfect – you just need plenty of practice. You know that the more unusual the sexual position you try, the higher the points you'll get. But you also get points for style and content and for sexual satisfaction, so you need to find a new position that works for both of you. Talk over the sexual positions you may have used to make love together – you may have tried woman-on-top, doggy style, standing up or you may not yet have ventured past man-on-top. Whatever, anything you've done so far is off limits now as being far too boring to earn points. Think about sexual positions you've heard about – standing, sitting, from behind, woman-on-top. You could also consider 69, with each of you giving the other oral sex, or trying it turn and turn about. You're about to start an hour-long training session, so get to it! You'll need a towel and energy drinks to keep you going through all that hot and sweaty work. You can use the dice to suggest parts of the body and actions to give you ideas, and the feather may tickle your fancies if the action flags. According to the *Kama Sutra*, there are eight basic positions for making love. Another ancient sex manual, *The Perfumed Garden*, says there are 11. What both agree is that there are literally hundreds of possible variations. You can ring eternal changes by shifting your bodies, bending or straightening legs, sitting up, leaning over, or supporting yourself on elbows, arms or

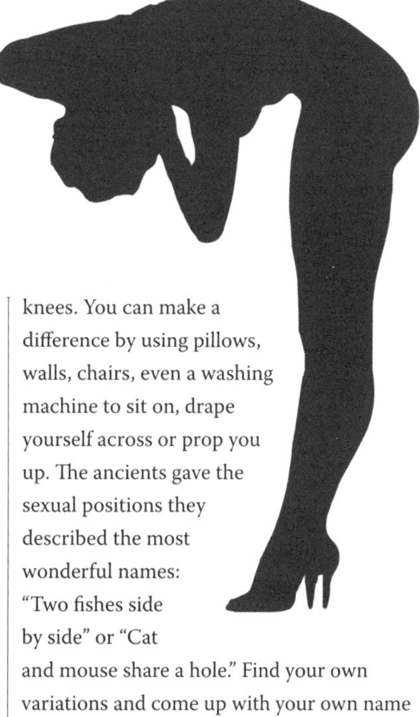

knees. You can make a difference by using pillows, walls, chairs, even a washing machine to sit on, drape yourself across or prop you up. The ancients gave the sexual positions they described the most wonderful names: "Two fishes side by side" or "Cat and mouse share a hole." Find your own variations and come up with your own name to describe them.

TOP TIP

Play Position of the Night when there is international gymnastics, athletics or ice skating on the television. Use the commentary, the marks and the applause as yours. Of course, when you're really experienced, try it to The Tour de France – all 14 days of it!

"13" Angels & Demons

He's a horny devil and she's an angel with an over-the-top innocent attitude – until he makes her his disciple!

Plunge the room into total darkness. She lies in bed as if asleep. He suddenly appears wearing nothing more than a tail and horns and a red silk cape, brandishing a pitchfork and ready to ravish her purity.

He jumps into bed and makes a grab for her. But just as he touches her, she runs away from him and hides. A hot and heavy game of hide-'n'-seek follows.

Virtue always triumphs over sin so she throws on the lights and takes charge, giving him a series of ultra good sexy deeds to do (to her) in order for him to find redemption – not to mention satisfaction!

Dress It Up

For Him:
* Red tail
* Red horns
* Red silk cape
* Pitchfork

For Her:
* Ultra-short floaty white dress
* Wings
* Halo
* Silver glitter
* White fishnet stockings
* Silver glitter heels
* Wand

Make It Real

He should use plenty of "bleeped" language. The more graphic he becomes in his descriptions of what he's going to do to her, the more she flinches, as if her oh-so-angelic innocence is being tarnished.

XXX Rating

Instead of a pitchfork, he can brandish a red dildo and use it as his devil's little helper.

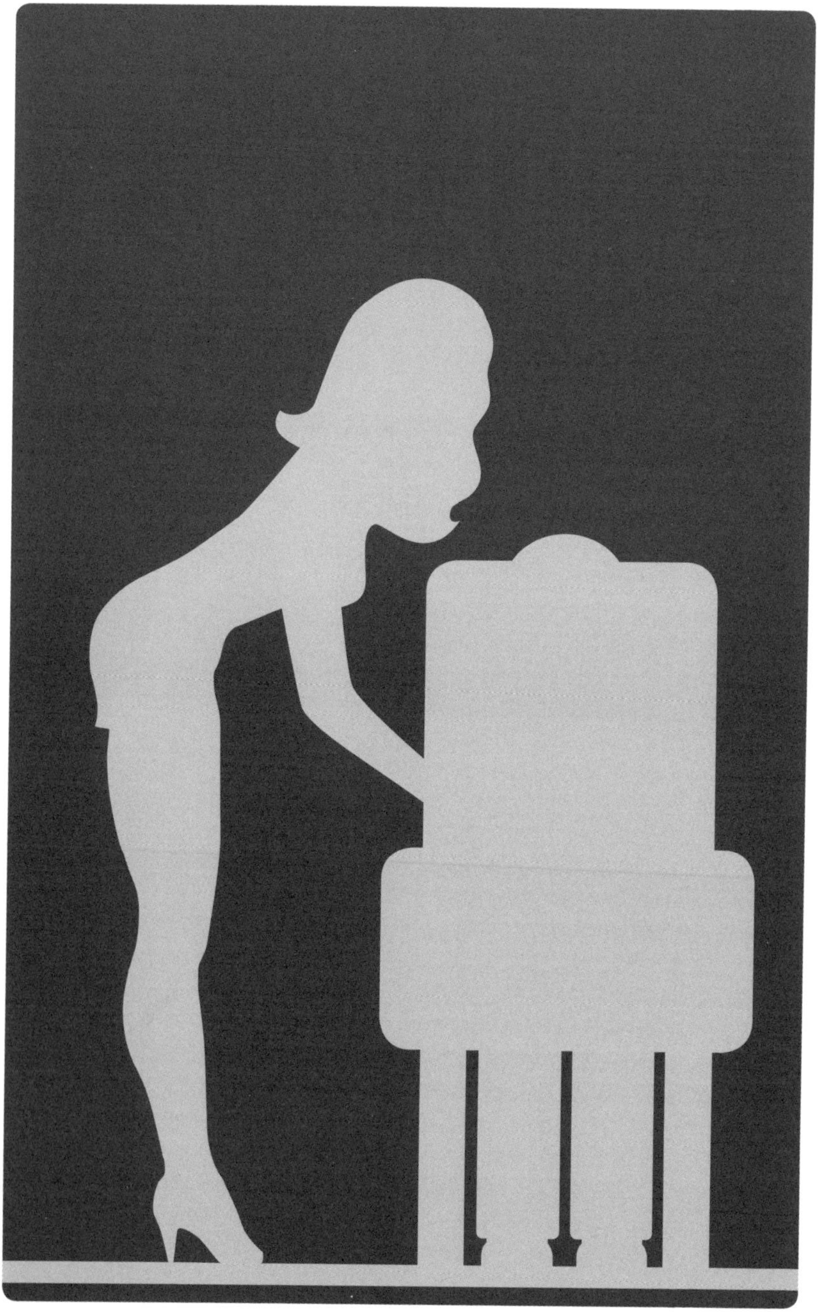

14
Prepare for Take-Off

There's a reason it's called a cockpit! You'll join the mile-high club when she dresses up as a sex-starved stewardess and he is the pleasure-seeking pilot.

Get ready for take-off by using a room in your home as the cockpit. Set up two padded chairs side by side in front of a window. He pretends to fly the plane and calls the stewardess to the cockpit, telling her that they will be experiencing turbulence. He then proceeds to tell her – explicitly – how to put his gear in a holding pattern.

Start with some in-flight entertainment. As the pilot is getting ready for take-off, she uses her hand or a vibrator to bring herself to cruising altitude.

Propel the scene along with some appropriate language. He asks her to come into the cockpit. She replies that she gets wet just hearing the word "cockpit" because she loves "cock" and begs him to say it again and again. He offers to show her his instrument panel and pulls out his "equipment," saying he has put the plane on autopilot and so they have time to do whatever they want.

Dress It Up

For Him:

* Pilot hat
* White short-sleeved shirt (add stripes to sleeves)
* Dark trousers
* Tie
* Airline wings badge

For Her:

* Mini-skirt and tight shirt in the same colour (preferably turquoise or pink)
* Wedge hat
* Scarf
* White go-go boots
* White gloves
* Airline wings brooch
* Small vibrator

Make It Real

Bring along a carry-on suitcase packed with travel accessories to make sure you have a smooth flight – miniature bottles of alcohol, small packets of snacks for eating off each other, a travel pillow and blanket, and hot steamy towels for cleaning up.

XXX Rating

Use the scarf or tie as a soft restraint.

⟪15⟫
Wild, Wild, Wild West

It's time to play Cowboys and Indians! If you don't have nosey neighbours, start your game outside. Otherwise, you can stalk each other in your house. Stealth and silence are all-important as she, dressed as an Indian, sneaks up on him, the Cowboy, and takes him captive by surprise. Once she has him prisoner, he begs for a peace powwow, during which he gives her everything she wants.

She refuses, saying he is in her power. She undresses him and ties him up, just tight enough so that he cannot escape. Should she scalp him, burn him at the stake or abandon him to fry under the hot sun? Instead, she removes a feather from her headdress and tickle-tortures him. Ever so slowly she drags the feather across his naked body until he screams for mercy.

For hardcore role-players, he overpowers her and, using his lasso, binds them together into a tight clinch to make wampum.

Dress It Up

For Him:
* Cowboy hat
* Leather cowboy boots
* Checked shirt
* Dungarees
* Bandana
* Fake gun or lasso

For Her:
* War paint
* Children's toy bow and arrows
* Headdress
* Leather fringed dress
* Moccasins

Make It Real

Finish by snuggling up in front of a campfire.

XXX Rating

She might not dare scalp him, but she can give him a close shave using a regular razor. He might return the favour, scalping a different part of her body.

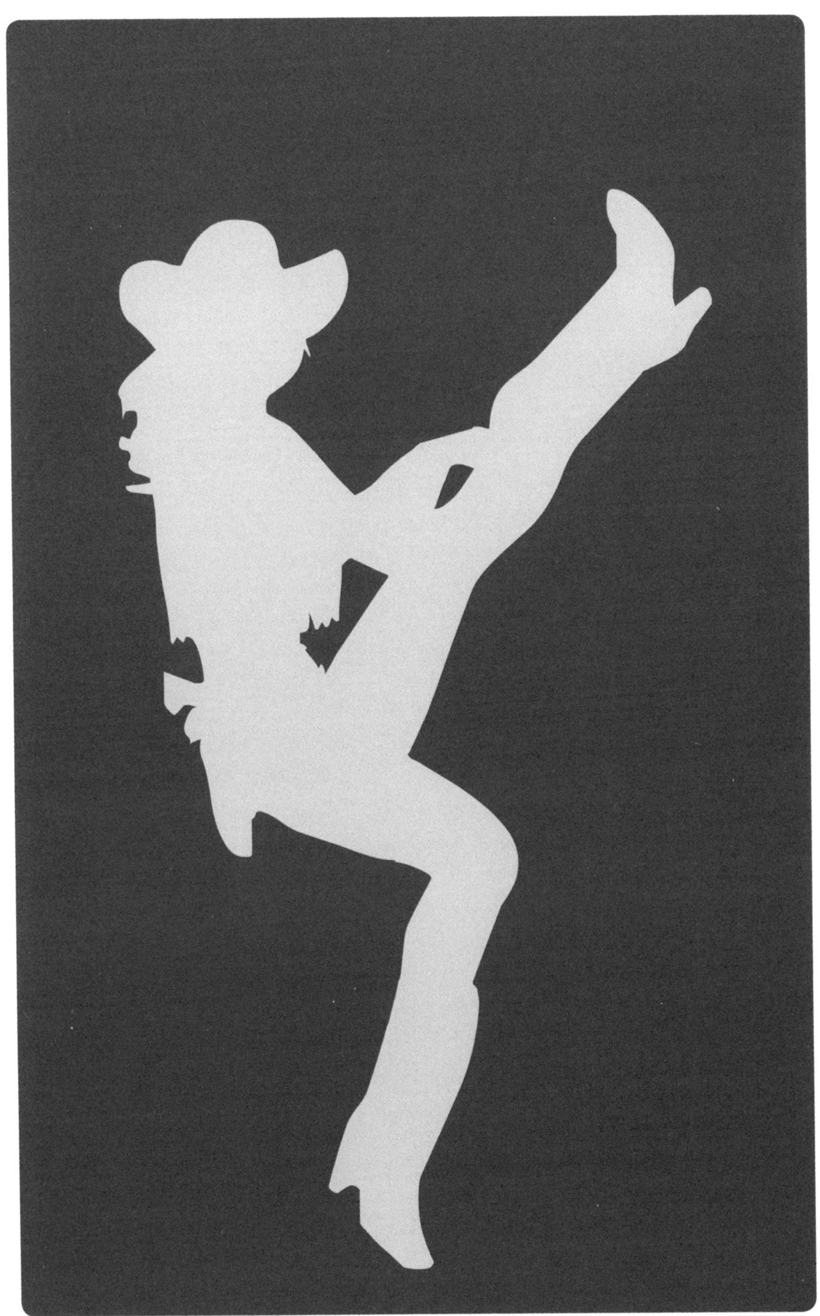

16
Hot Cop

What will you do to get out of this speeding ticket? He sits in "the driver's seat." She saunters up in her raunchy cop's uniform, ready to throw the book at him. He offers to do anything to avoid getting ticketed. She takes him up on his offer, telling him to "spread 'em."

He runs to avoid arrest. She gives chase, catching him in the bedroom. She sternly tells him he is being arrested for carrying a deadly weapon, cuffs his hands behind his back and reads him his rights. She then plays with his "gun" until it "accidentally" goes off.

Who's been a naughty boy? That's right: someone needs a lesson in police procedure! Designate an area as the "cells." She leads her "prisoner" there. Thrilling to the idea that he is under her control, she tells him he is entirely in her hands – there's no calling his lawyer this time! She removes his belt and shoelaces and then strip-searches him. Because he is a deviant criminal, she decides to keep him in solitary confinement until he serves his time.

Dress It Up

For Him:
* Belted trousers
* Shoes with laces

For Her:
* Cop's hat
* Sexy police uniform
* Fake gun/night stick
* Handcuffs
* Ticket book
* Police sunglasses
* Shield

Make It Real

She politely refers to him as "Sir" the entire time and keeps her voice deadpan.

XXX Rating

In the ticket book, she can write various "punishments" – 20 minutes of lip service, a one-hour rub down, receiver's choice and so on…

"17"
Starring Role

It's movie night! Send yourselves an invitation to a costume party. You and your guest are asked to wear matching costumes. But it's a week before Halloween and all the costumes have been picked through. You have no choice but to go as (insert favourite movie personalities). Once you are geared up, act out your top movie scenes with these characters – then rewrite the scripts to include an especially exciting climax.

Alternatively, challenge yourselves to a weekend of living as your characters. Or throw a costume party yourselves. Mid-revelry, slip off to act out your own thrilling adventure – just make sure you grab the right character to rehearse with!

Dress It Up
* Hans Solo and Princess Leia
* Batman and Catwoman
* Superman and Wonder Woman
* Captain Kirk or Picard and a female Klingon or Vulcan (how can you tell?)
* Tarzan and Jane

Make It Real
Use actual scripts from the movies (www. imsdb.com is a good source for loads of free online scripts).

XXX Rating
Instead of getting the actual costume, splash out for the sex shop versions, which will have handy openings and come with titillating accessories such as a vibrating light sabre or a leather cat-o-nine tails.

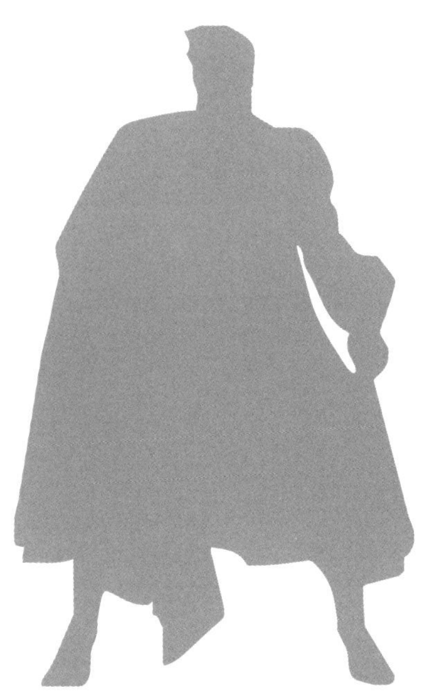

❝18❞
Roman Romp

Take a trip back to ancient Rome for a night of decadent loving. Begin your orgy of pleasure by planning to while away the day in the bath. Fill the tub with warm water and mix in a cupful of scented oil. Take it in turns to soak in the perfumed water or, if the tub is big enough, bathe together. Make it a really sensual experience, languorously washing every inch of your partner's body with large sponges soaked alternately in hot and cold water. Feed each other grapes and drink large goblets of wine. Once you are completely clean, ravage each other dirty again.

Slather yourselves in oil and nude-wrestle. The loser gives the winner some thumb's up action.

Slip into a toga (nothing underneath, obviously). Drape it so that all it takes is a simple tug to hail each other's Caesar. See how many positions you can do reclining on a bed of cushions.

Dress It Up

For Him:

* Sheet for toga
* Vine crown
* Simple leather sandals

For Her:

* Jewels to wear in her hair
* Sheet for toga
* Small tiara
* Simple leather sandals

Make It Real

Once dressed, indulge in a great feast. Romans ate their meals while lolling on couches (slaves sat at the table, ready to "serve"). Make sure there is plenty of fresh fruit – peaches, pineapples, pomegranates, passion fruit, figs and, of course, juicy grapes – to feed each other.

XXX Rating

Turn it into a feast of pleasure – eat food from one another's body, try passing the wine from one mouth to another without spilling a drop, or catch grapes in your mouths (if you miss, you perform a forfeit).

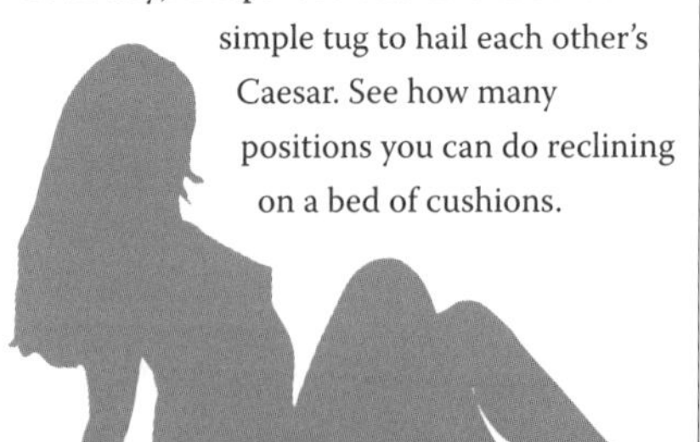

19
Express Service

She has a crush on the delivery man and has been dying to check out his package. He usually leaves the boxes and knocks on the door before he gets back in his truck and drives away. This time she plans to catch him and seduce him. She dresses in her sexiest lingerie. When he drives up, she tells him she has a tip and invites him in. She closes the door and gives him some lip service.

He tells her he has a route to finish. She says that she doesn't care and that she has a special parcel for him. Slipping out of her lingerie, she strikes a seductive pose and asks him if he thinks he can deliver. To heat things up, tell him that it's an express service and he has five minutes to wrap things up.

Dress It Up

For Him:

✳ Any sort of delivery outfit will do

✳ A box or two (see Make It Real)

For Her:

✳ Skimpy lingerie

Make It Real

Order up some sex toys by post about a week before you plan to play. Don't open the box when it arrives – he can use it as his prop when he makes his delivery.

XXX Rating

Tear open your package and use what's inside to send each other to orgasm island.

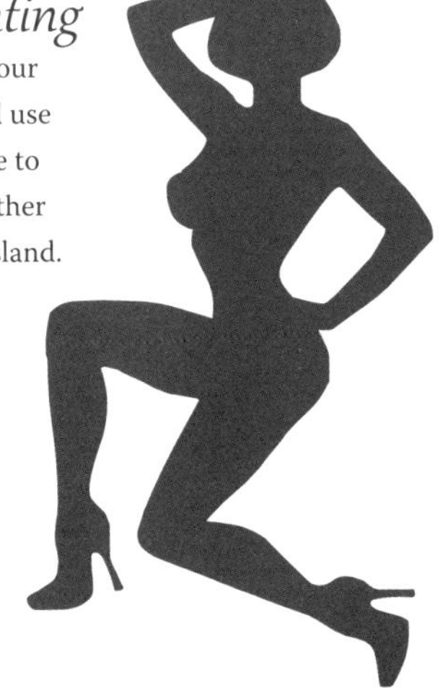

"20
Artistic Vision

One of you is an artist or a photographer creating a piece of art from the other's nude model. Don't worry about having any talent. This is just an excuse to study your lover long and hard. The artist sets up their sketch pad and instructs the model to pose exactly how they want. They can do whatever they want with the model for "art's sake," telling them how to stand and pose with whatever props you have to hand.

The artist tells their model to play with themselves, saying that they want to sketch their orgasm.

Switch to video and keep the camera running even after you live up to your randy reputations as artistic types and make wild beautiful love on the studio floor.

Dress It Up

For Him:

✳ Loose white shirt

✳ Baggy trousers

For Her:

✳ Black shirt

✳ Black leggings

Make It Real

Lighting is incredibly important. Keep it low and flattering to avoid looking like you are making Art Attack or Vincent Van Grow (unless that is the storyline you are creating).

XXX Rating

Experiment with different positions that leave nothing to the imagination.

21
Down & Dirty, Ooh La La

Turn housework into play time with a little je ne sais quoi and a frisky French outfit.

She goes into the bedroom before him and starts lightly dusting the furniture. When he comes in a few moments later, she says in a French accent, "Oh, s'il vous plaît, so sorry, I was given permission to take extra time to do an extra special job." She then looks him over and says, "Pardon, monsieur, your clothes are so dirtee. Let me remove them for you." Before long, the door handles are not the only knobs she is polishing.

Alternatively, he doesn't wait for her to give him a rub down. Being a good servant, she doesn't protest when he throws her on the bed and takes her. Still playing the sub (submissive), she offers to wash him down in the shower afterwards.

Turn the tables, and zut alors, she is a saucy French maid who ties her master to the bed and teases him with a feather duster for leaving his socks on the floor.

Dress It Up
For Him:
✳ Something elegant such as a suit and tie or a tux

For Her:
✳ Short black dress, usually with a lacy or fluffy crinoline underneath and white trim
✳ Small white apron
✳ Tiny hat
✳ Black seamed stockings

Make It Real
Speak your lines in ze French accent.

XXX Rating
Take your action out of the house – rent a hotel room to play in.

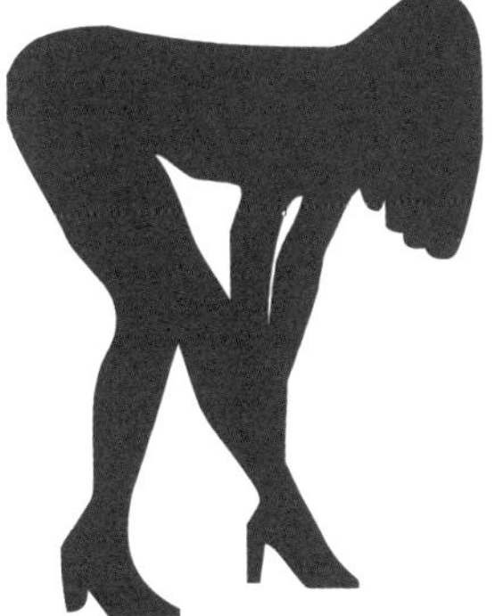

~22~
Happily Ever After

Who doesn't dream of a fairy-tale ending to the randy rendezvous?

Sleeping Beauty is in a deep sleep so she lies down on the bed (a couch will also do), with her eyes closed. Along comes Prince Charming, ready to rescue her. He knows a simple kiss will just not be enough to break the spell and awaken her. Kneeling down beside her, he opens her bodice and bra and then lightly caresses her chest to make sure she is still breathing. He continues to work his way down, down, down, stroking her body with his fingers. He slides down her knickers and, spreading her legs, rubs her treasure spot until she begins to moan. His princess is awake.

Sleeping Beauty opens her eyes and breathes, "My Prince!" She sees the bulge between his legs and invites him to release his royal sabre.

Dress It Up

For Him:
* Crown
* Breeches or leggings
* Velvet purple or burgundy cape
* White silky, blousy shirt
* (Fake) sword
* High boots

For Her:
* Silky gown that opens at the front
* Slippers
* Crown
* Sexy bra and underwear

Make It Real

Study the fairy tale and use actual language from the plot.

XXX Rating

Instead of awakening her with a caress, Prince Charming brings Sleeping Beauty back to life with a kiss to her nether regions.

"23"
Bedroom Idol

It's your lucky night as your favourite Hollywood hottie of the moment (or a hunka-hunka fusion of as many celebs as you lust for) makes a star appearance in your bed.

Your star sweetie is making a movie and you have a backstage pass. You sneak into their trailer (your bedroom) and, taking off your clothes, lie in wait as a guest surprise.

Instead of a Hollywood icon, your celeb is a top-tier porn star. You play out scenes from their most hardcore off-the-wall, on-the-couch, under-the-bed, in-the-restroom, up-a-tree, on-a-car action. (Check online for the top 100 adult films of all time at www.gamelink.com.)

Dress It Up

If you are the celeb, check out a gossip mag for inspiration

If you are the star-struck groupie, everyday clothes will do

Make It Real

Re-enact a sex scene that your dream lover has actually played in.

XXX Rating

Log onto www.celebritysexfantasy.com for adult movies starring your favourite lookalike celebs.

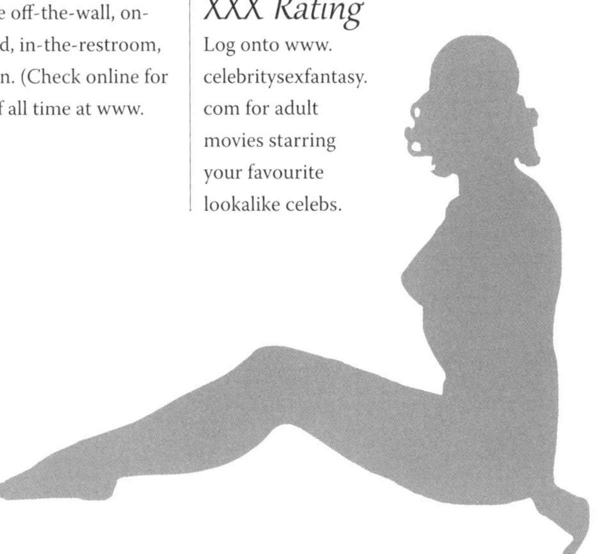

"24" Close-Ups

Get inspired by cinema's hottest love scenes. The movie scenes women find most exciting deal with emotional connection and gazing into each other's eyes, while men get off on the ones where they can see some skin. Here are seven that work for both:

The Big Easy The awkward stop-and-start pacing and preference for dialogue over heavy breathing will please her while Ellen Barkin's orgasm will satisfy him.

Titanic She'll get hot and bothered by the doomed young couple love story while he'll appreciate Kate Winslet showing how to make a rumble seat really rumble.

Shakespeare in Love She'll be primed from literary love while he will be Gwyneth Paltrow's Bard-core moment.

Thelma and Louise Her heart will be stolen by Brad Pitt – and so will his.

Bull Durham You'll both make a home-run as a pedicure turns into a passionate treatment in full-body sex.

Ghost She'll get horny weeping over doomed love while his artistic side will appreciate some messy, clay-covered sex.

Stealing Beauty You'll both play and replay the scene where Liv Tyler loses her virginity to a sexy young Italian boy.

The best movie sex depends on the surprise, the strangeness, the thrilling newness of a steamy encounter out of your usual environs. These seven impromptu hot-and-heavy interludes will all tap your risqué, reckless feeling of "We might get caught, but who cares?" exhibitionist streak.

1 The kitchen sink moment in *Fatal Attraction*
2 Against the wall in *Sea of Love*
3 In the restaurant bathroom in *Unfaithful*
4 On a train in *Risky Business*
5 Halfway up the stairs in *A History of Violence* (bonus moment: teenage cheerleading role-play sex)
6 In a limo (or car) in *No Way Out*
7 In the pool, at the carwash (is there anywhere these three don't do it?) in *Wild Things*

On-screen sex scenes tend to get really hot when they depict something kinky. Five movies to ring your raunch bell:

1 *Something Wild* breaks out the handcuffs but he can loosely tie her wrists with a silk or velvet scarf if you don't want to bond under lock and key.
2 *Last Tango in Paris* uses butter but you can feed your fantasies with any food or even an ice cube.
3 *Body of Evidence* shows what else candles are good for besides providing romantic lighting.
4 *Basic Instinct* is a primer in how to flash a roomful of men – or just that special someone – without catching a draught.
5 *Emmanuelle* will spur you on to put your sexual fantasies to good use.

Dress It Up

Use the film as your inspiration for how you dress.

Make It Real

Set an Oscar-worthy scene – movie sex is orchestrated to the very last detail. You don't have to redecorate but you can tidy up to create a high-octane erotic charge in your home. None of Keira Knightley's characters would make love in a bedroom cluttered with bills, a Thighmaster and photos of your cat, and neither should you. Boudoir staples really do work – satin sheets, flickering candles and filmy curtains swirling in the breeze (much sexier than miniblinds). Same goes for whatever room you end up in – surrounding the bath with candles, dimming the lighting in the lounge or cleaning the remnants of dinner off the dining table will give your scene star quality.

XXX Rating

Some of the raciest sex scenes come from the chemistry of a clean-cut guy and a bossy vixen revved up and ready to roll into bed. Even if you are not hardwired to act like this, there are plenty of little ways to unleash the sex symbol within and leave him feeling blissfully ravished – you can flirt with him, using girlie moves like twirling your hair or stroking your neck, or pull a "helpless little me" move and ask for his help putting on your bra and shirt. Or use sound effects with lots of groans, moans, sighs and take-me-now's.

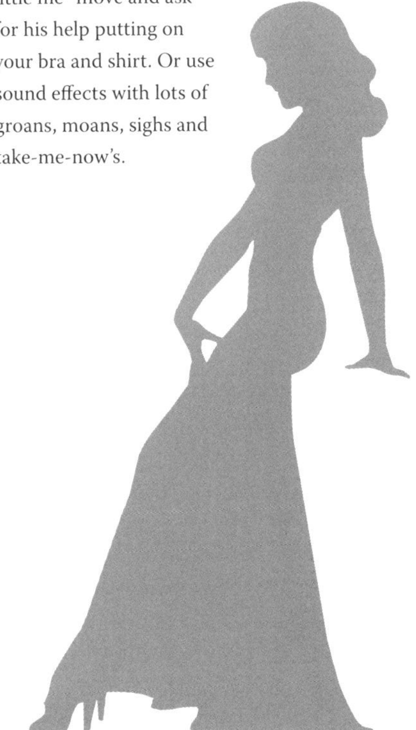

"25"
Royal Moments

She is a damsel in distress, running away from her evil stepmother queen. He is her knight in shining armour.

Turn your home into a castle by draping lots of cloth and tapestry around. She bangs on the front door, looking to escape the horsemen who have been ordered to kill her. He lets her in and, seeing that she is chilled, begins to rub her down. Gradually, he heats her up to the point where she loses her royal composure.

Seeing that time is of the essence, he tells her to jump on his steed and he will take her away. She sits on his lap and they ride at a fast pace.

He is in cahoots with her stepmother. He brings her "down" to his dungeon, which is kitted out in instruments of torture (handcuffs, light whip, nipple clamps, etc). He turns her into his sex slave.

Dress It Up

For Him:
* High boots
* (Fake) sword
* Snood
* Vest
* Leggings

For Her:
* Gown
* Crown

Make It Real

He can invest in a chain-mail tunic, available from costume supply stores.

XXX Rating

Doubting her purity, he can put a chastity belt on her.

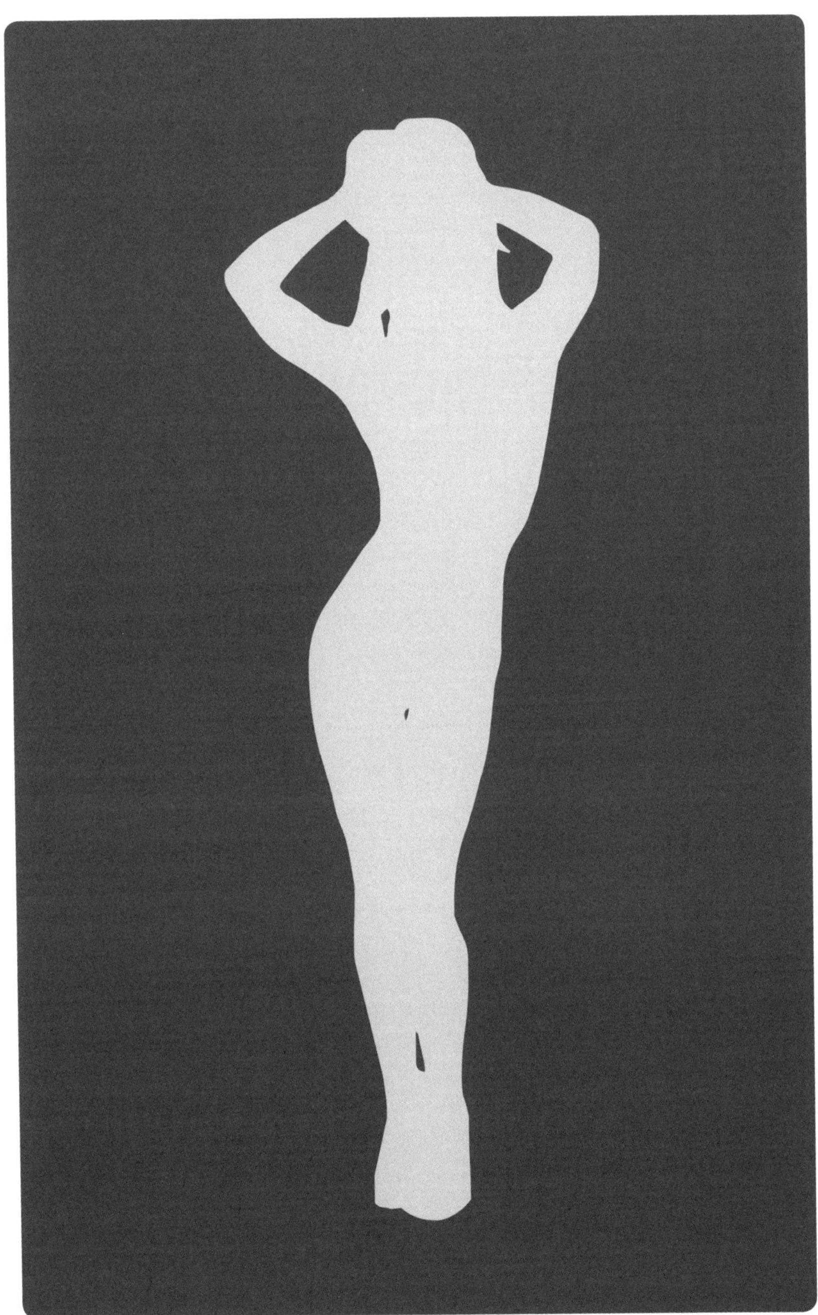

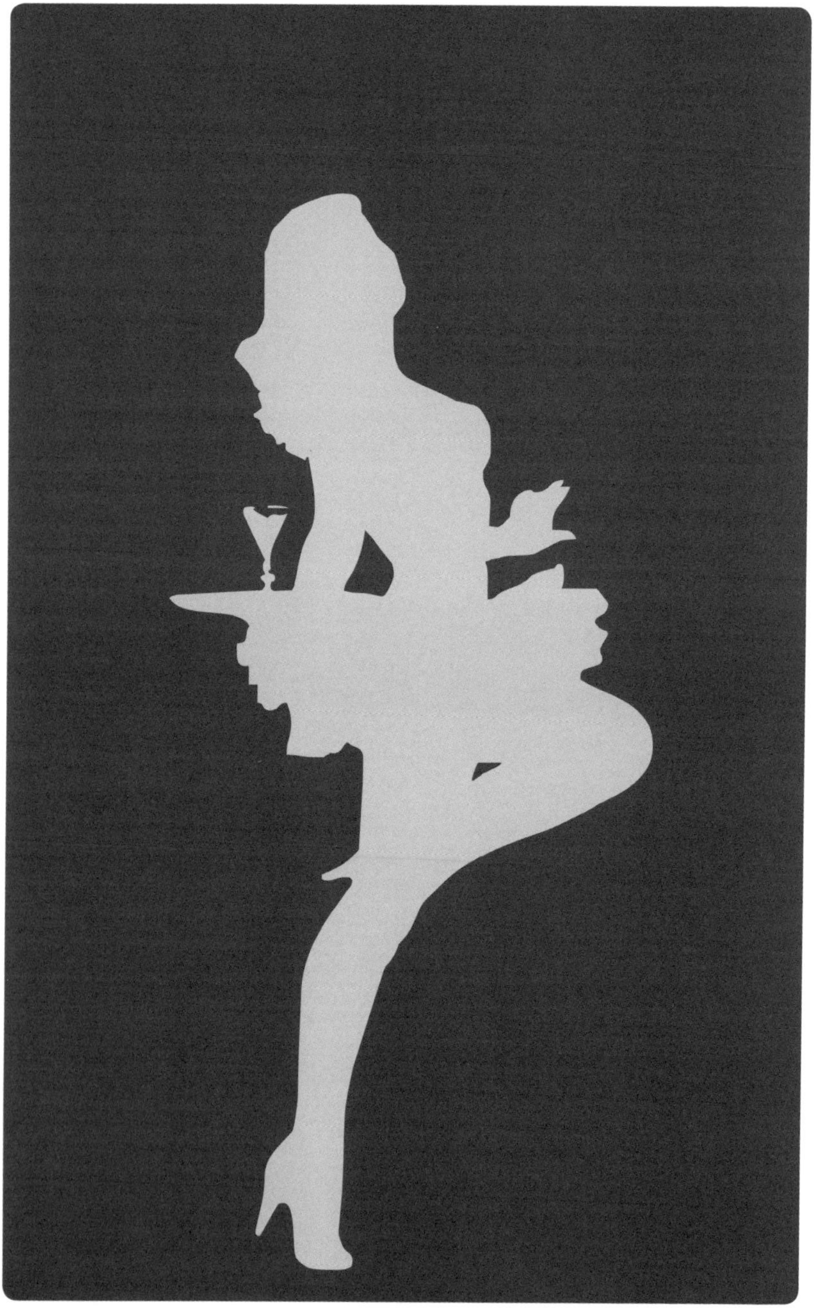

26 Coffee, Tea or Me?

Get ready to serve up some passion on a platter when she dresses up as a full-service hostess with the mostess. Have a table set. When he arrives, he should greet her by her waitress name (it's written on a badge on her shirt). She seats him at a candlelit table covered in a crisp white tablecloth. She places a napkin on his lap, carefully smoothing it down and making sure it covers everything. She then begins to recite the night's specials, such as a two-minute lap dance, a back massage, a mini striptease or a full-body massage. She asks if he wants a tasting menu or if he wants to order à la carte. Create a menu of fun and flirty treats your partner can try.

The customer is always right so he gets to order special off-menu items. Her tip will be based on how well she "serves" them.

She turns him into the plat du jour. She covers his chest and all the way down and around his penis with whipped cream and not-too-hot fudge. Then she places strawberries randomly over his chest and slowly eats each one before licking the sticky sauces off.

Dress It Up

For Him:

✳ Evening clothes

For Her:

✳ A short plain black dress

✳ A frilly white apron

✳ A lacy headscarf or hanky for a hat

Make It Real

She should serve up some sensual foods to feed him:

✳ Grapes

✳ Bananas

✳ Champagne

✳ Strawberries

✳ Chocolate

✳ Oysters

✳ Whipped cream

XXX Rating

She can serve him nyotaimori, or "naked sushi." She lies naked with sushi adorning her body, which he then eats directly off her.

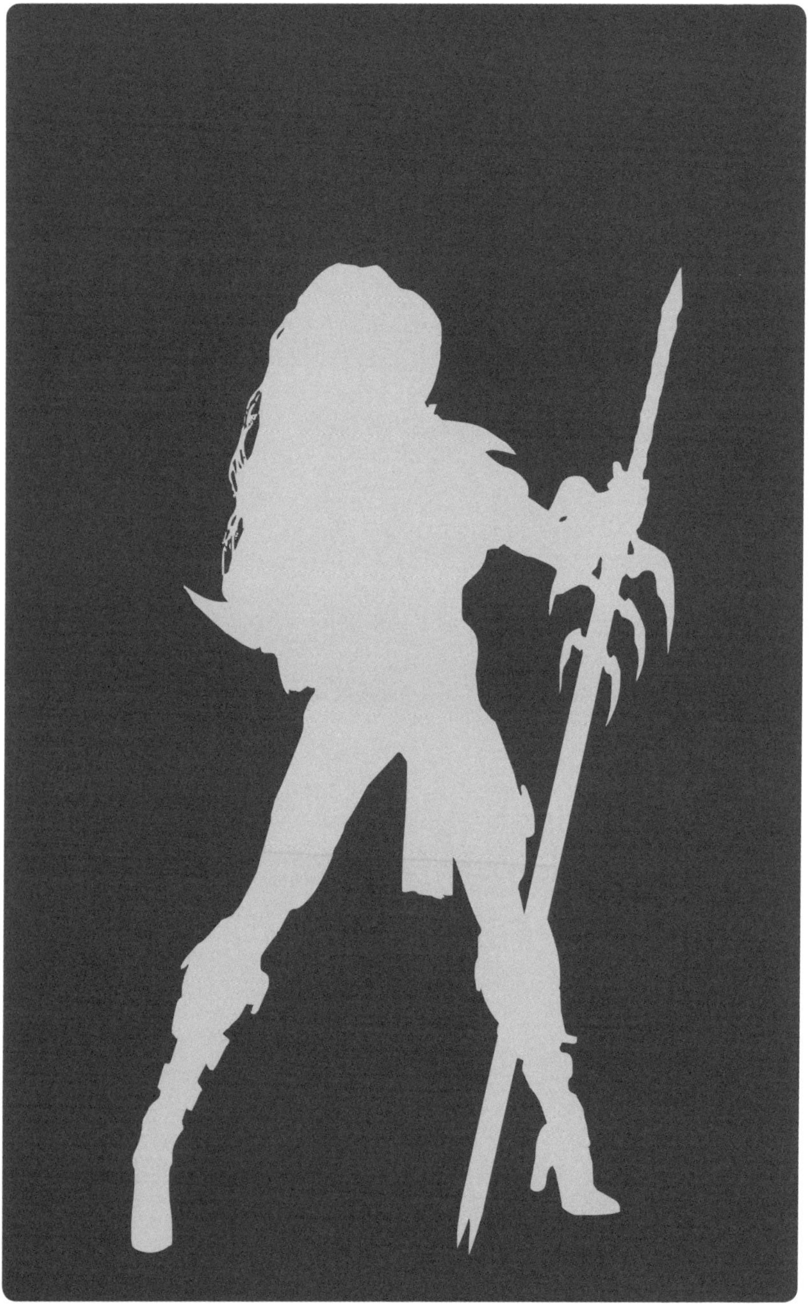

27
Virtual Orgasms

Different from porn, which is all about the money, cyber games are a risk-free way of flirting with different randy roles using your computer.

In the world of erotic video games, there are loads of virtual sex games and they all treat it a little differently, but here are some steps, tips and tricks to get you started. You'll need a disk-based game, computer, downloaded game file and major console

Find a site that intrigues you. The biggest are Sims (www.thesims2.ea.com), Sociolotron SM (www.sociolotron.amerabyte.com), Playskins (www.playskins.com) and Second Life (www.secondlife.com). Each online role-playing game (RPG) is a bit different – some are all about the sex; others just include sex. Test out a few before you commit (some have monthly fees that allow you to play for a while and quit if you do not like them). In some games, nudity and sexual behaviour are forbidden outside private areas and sex clubs.

Next, create your character, then get yourself familiar with your virtual universe by learning the rules of the game and the conventions of game play. You can sit back and observe to see how others interact and build on their models. Start making virtual friends. You'll soon find a character that you click with. Make some nano nookie. Use suggestive language to segue into virtual sex, and then proceed with whatever the game allows.

If you're experienced with virtual sex games, don't just chat about sex. You can buy outfits to dress your avatars provocatively, or "skins" to make them appear nude. In some games, you may also need to purchase your avatar's genitals. Once you have the look and voice of your avatar down, buy equipment, ranging from realistic-looking beds and other furniture to fanciful torture devices used in BDSM fantasies.

Dress It Up

You can be as dressed or undressed as you desire.

Make It Real

Be extremely wary of meeting in real life anybody you encounter online. This is especially true if you met them in a virtual sex game.

XXX Rating

Have real sex virtually – guys can get a virtual sex stroker for the penis while cyber babes can try out the virtual vibrator.

~28~
Who's the Boss?

He has an important assignment for her – to pleasure him. He's behind the desk, talking on the phone. She's the temp, working in the other room, on the computer. He sends her an email saying he needs her assistance right away. When she comes in, she finds that he's unzipped his trousers and has an erection. He tells her she has a five-minute deadline to bring him off.

She hides underneath the boss's big desk before the start of an "important meeting." Slowly – and very quietly – she performs oral sex on him with the clients sitting right there. His challenge? To keep a straight face and continue with his meeting. Alternatively, he may be on the phone and has to continue with his phone conversation without faltering.

For hardcore role-players, take the above action to his actual place of work.

Dress It Up
For Him:
* Suit
* Shirt
* Tie

For Her:
* Prim skirt
* Blouse
* Sensible shoes
* Tights

Make It Real

Threaten to bring him up on sexual harassment charges – that is, if he doesn't give you a pay rise!

XXX Rating
He gives you very suggestive dictation.

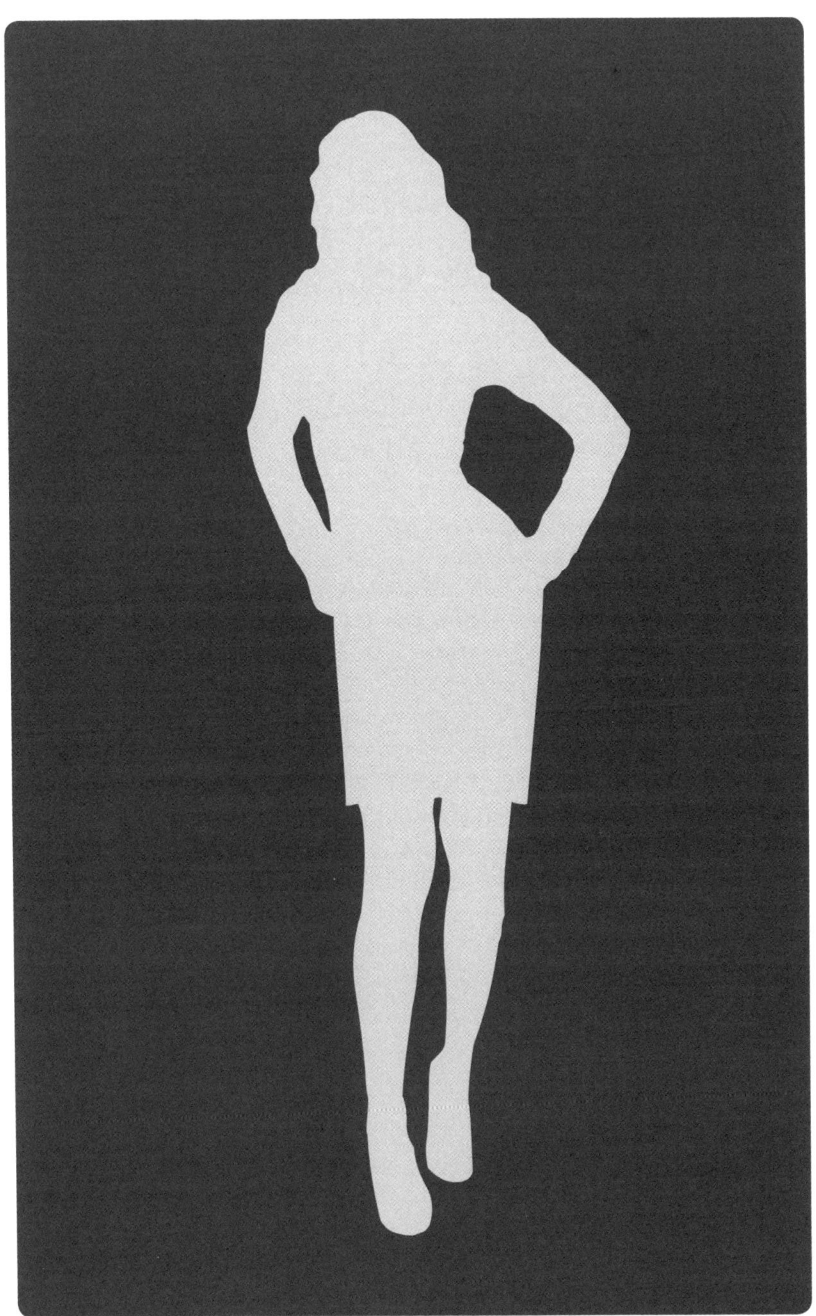

29
Kidnapped Victim

She's a wealthy bluest-of-blood duchess abducted by a rakish highwayman who demands sex instead of money as ransom. She is taking some air out in the garden and doesn't see him coming. He sneaks up behind and slips a blindfold over her eyes and, using a scarf/rope/handcuffs, ties her arms behind her back. He says that she is now under his control and marches her into the bedroom. He unties her. Whispering dirty words in her ear, he begins to seduce her, running his hands up and down her clothed body, undressing her hurriedly. You finish with wild sex.

He reties her hands so they are now above her head/attached to the bedposts. He then proceeds to tease and torment her body until she is straining against her bonds and begging him to take her now.

For hardcore role-players, as he brings her to the bedroom, she struggles and tells him she will never succumb, no matter what he does to her. He ties her bottom up on the bed and proceeds to lightly spank her. He asks if she will be a good girl. She meekly promises to do anything he wants as long as he doesn't hurt her.

Dress It Up

For Him:

* White shirt open to navel
* Some sort of fake weapon
* High boots
* Three-day beard

For Her:

* Long gown with lots of buttons

Make It Real

She should try and speak in an uppercrust accent, while he can use more common language. In the end, as in all the best historical romances, she should fall in love with him.

XXX Rating

Keep the blindfold on.

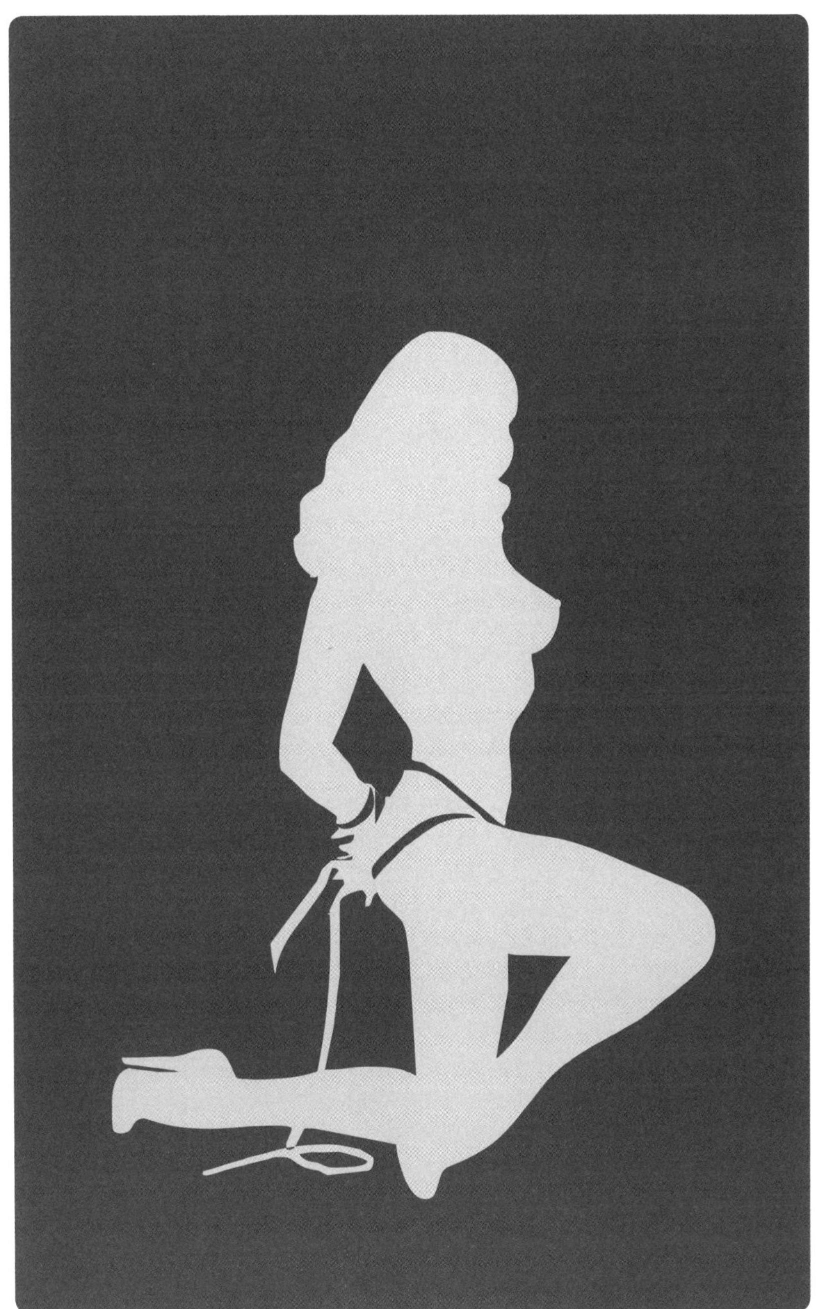

"30"
No! No! Oh Yes! Yessssss!

In this favourite female fantasy, he takes her against her will. She is alone in her bedroom, naked. He sneaks up behind her, covers her eyes and mouth and says, "I won't hurt you if you do everything I say." She's helpless as he takes his hand from her eyes and explores and strokes her body. He challenges her to tell him she is not enjoying what he is doing. Sigh. She can't.

Coming to her senses, she tries to escape. They wrestle. He grabs her by the hair, pulls her arms behind her back, and forces her head down to his crotch. He unzips and orders her to take care of him.

Dress It Up

For Him:

✳ Street clothes

For Her:

✳ Birthday suit

Make It Real

She wants to feel completely overpowered so

he should be as forceful as he can without actually hurting her – running his fingers through her hair and pulling, nibbling roughly at her skin, ripping her clothes without care.

XXX Rating

Because this involves a lot of unbridled force, before you start, set up a code word to stop the action if it gets too much.

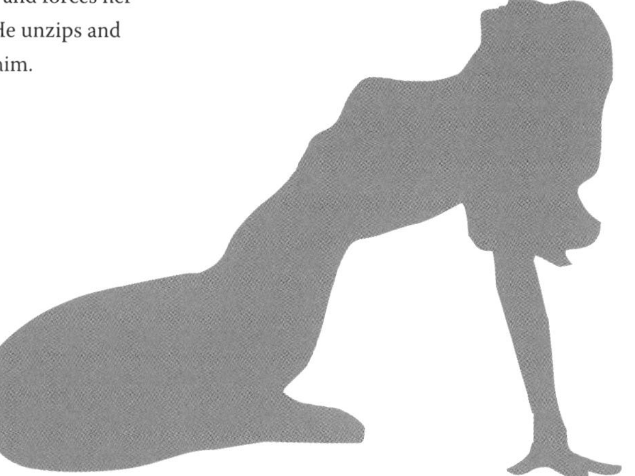